"In my candidacy at the White Institute in the early fifties, I was interviewed by Dr. Thompson, took her courses, was in supervision with her and later came to know her during summers on the Cape. I am delighted to see this thoughtful and respectful book by Dr. D'Ercole. It is a labor of love by a prominent feminist psychoanalyst in tribute to a much-overlooked major contributor to psychoanalytic theory and practice. That is, of course, consistent with the treatment of women in most scientific venues at the time, but also 'Clara's' (we all called her that, but not always to her face) modesty led her to act as a portal to the work of Sullivan and Fromm—the two other founders of WAW. Dr. D'Ercole has done an outstanding job of explicating Dr. Thompson's prescient contributions to modern psychoanalytic theory and practice but has also grasped her in her most human aspects. For all my long association with Dr. Thompson, and in spite of her friendliness and egalitarianism, I hardly knew her. I trust this outstanding book will remedy this oversight and revitalize a much-deserved interest in this most interesting and complex person."

Edgar Levenson is a fellow emeritus, faculty, training, supervisory analyst at the William Alanson White Institute; he is adjunct clinical professor of Psychology at New York University, and author of *Fallacy of Understanding; The Ambiguity of Change; The Purloined Self;* and *Interpersonal Psychoanalysis and the Enigma of Consciousness*

"Clara Thompson was not only one of the most important leaders in the psychoanalysis of her time, but also one of the singular figures in the entire history of the discipline. She was a pioneer in so many ways, founding and then directing one of the most significant psychoanalytic institutes, bringing together the work of Erich Fromm and Harry Stack Sullivan to create interpersonal psychoanalysis, and creating one of the first bodies of work devoted to the psychology of women. She was one of those who created the study of gender and sexuality. She was a powerfully inspiring leader at a time when that was highly unusual for a woman in psychiatry or psychoanalysis. Thompson richly deserves Ann D'Ercole's deep, thorough, and moving account of her life. This two-volume work is absolutely riveting, an instant classic that will be read and studied not only by psychoanalysts and other psychotherapists, but by anyone interested in cultural history, feminism, the history of psychiatry, and gender and sexuality."

Donnel Stern most recently authored *The Infinity of the Unsaid: Unformulated Experience, Language, and the Nonverbal*

"Ann D'Ercole's two-volume biography carefully documents and reveals Clara Thompson's often-overlooked role and contributions to the development of interpersonal psychoanalysis in the United States. 'Clara,' as interpersonalists still refer to her today, was analyzed by Sándor Ferenczi in Budapest and worked closely with Harry Stack Sullivan, Erich Fromm and Frieda Fromm-Reichman. She was the first Director of the William Alanson White Institute in New York City (currently housed in the Clara Thompson building) and the training and supervising analyst for many pioneers of contemporary interpersonal and relational theory. D'Ercole has done an exemplary and engaging job of correcting this historical omission of Thompson's foundational role as 'An American Psychoanalyst.'"

Jack Drescher is a training and supervising analyst at the William Alanson White Institute; adjunct professor of the Postdoctoral Program in Psychotherapy and Psychoanalysis; a clinical professor of Psychiatry at Columbia University; and senior psychoanalytic consultant at the Columbia Center for Psychoanalytic Training and Research

"Ann D'Ercole has accomplished a special scholarly work about Clara Thompson, M.D. Has Thompson having been a foremost student of Sándor Ferenczi placed her in the analytic shadows? Ann's thorough, lively and insightful writing brings Thompson out of the shadows and into the limelight where she belongs. Ann's outstanding research has clarified Thompson's brilliant contributions to psychoanalysis: a prominent figure in establishing the American School of Psychoanalysis; a leading contributor in the formation of the Interpersonal School of Psychoanalysis; a leading student and advocate of the work of Sándor Ferenczi and Henry Stack Sullivan; a founder of the William Alanson White Institute; a leading feminist of her time; a pioneering theorist and clinician in establishing the two person perspective in psychoanalysis. Ann's biography of Thompson should become the premium resource that rediscovers the importance of Clara Thompson for psychoanalysis."

Arnold Wm. Rachman is a Training and Supervisory Analyst, Postgraduate Psychoanalytic Institute, NYC; Clinical Professor of Psychology, Adelphi University Postdoctoral Program in Psychoanalysis and Psychotherapy, Garden City, NY; Associate Professor of Psychiatry, New York University Medical Center, NYC; Donor, Elizabeth Severn Papers, The Library of Congress; recent publication - *Psychoanalysis and Society's Neglect of the Sexual Abuse of Children, Youth and Adults,* Routledge

"In this engaging paean to the life of Clara Thompson, D'Ercole excavates, brings to life, and carries forth the historical record in adroitly making the case that Thompson deserves placement in the upper echelons of the pantheon of psychoanalysts. She plumbs the depths of her own personal connection to Thompson in illuminating the essential contributions of Thompson to the field of interpersonal psychoanalysis. A hidden gem, not just for readers unfamiliar with Thompson's work, this is a must read for all."

Jean Petrucelli is faculty, training, and supervising analyst at the William Alanson White Institute; adjunct professor and clinical consultant of the NYU Postdoctoral Program in Psychotherapy and Psychoanalysis; and most recently, co-editor of the book, *Patriarchy and Its Discontents*

Clara M. Thompson's Professional Evolution and Legacy

Beginning in 1933, after Sándor Ferenczi's death, this volume draws extensively from interviews, personal correspondence, and scholarly essays to explore the latter part of Clara Thompson's life and professional career.

The reader is afforded an understanding of Thompson's development with the luminaries who influenced her, and who she, in turn, influenced, including Harry Stack Sullivan, Erich Fromm, and other "cultural" social scientists. Building on her collaborative work with Ferenczi, and influenced by Sullivan, Thompson's pioneering essays expand the psychoanalytic perspective to embrace the dynamic interpersonal encounter between patient and analyst. Critical of Freud's views on women, Thompson also argues against the inequality of women and men in society, reflecting her own moral compass. This volume clarifies Thompson's role in psychoanalytic history, reclaiming her numerous and valuable contributions to both the interpersonal psychoanalytic tradition and to the field of psychoanalysis as we know it today.

D'Ercole's artfully woven account of Thompson's life will prove essential reading for psychoanalysts, psychotherapists, psychologists, and anyone interested in the history of psychoanalysis.

Ann D'Ercole is a Clinical Associate Professor of Psychology at the New York University Postdoctoral Program in Psychotherapy and Psychoanalysis, where she is both teaching faculty and supervisor. She is also a distinguished visiting faculty at the William Alanson White Institute and recipient of the APA, Division 39, Sexualities and Gender Identities Award for Outstanding Contributions to the Advancement of Sexualities and Gender Identities in Psychoanalysis. Dr. D'Ercole is in private practice in New York City.

Psychoanalysis in A New Key Book Series
Donnel Stern
Series Editor

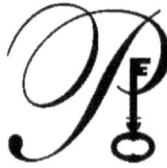

When music is played in a new key, the melody does not change, but the notes that make up the composition do: change in the context of continuity, continuity that perseveres through change. Psychoanalysis in a New Key publishes books that share the aims psychoanalysts have always had, but that approach them differently. The books in the series are not expected to advance any particular theoretical agenda, although to this date most have been written by analysts from the Interpersonal and Relational orientations.

The most important contribution of a psychoanalytic book is the communication of something that nudges the reader's grasp of clinical theory and practice in an unexpected direction. Psychoanalysis in a New Key creates a deliberate focus on innovative and unsettling clinical thinking. Because that kind of thinking is encouraged by exploration of the sometimes surprising contributions to psychoanalysis of ideas and findings from other fields, Psychoanalysis in a New Key particularly encourages interdisciplinary studies. Books in the series have married psychoanalysis with dissociation, trauma theory, sociology, and criminology. The series is open to the consideration of studies examining the relationship between psychoanalysis and any other field—for instance, biology, literary and art criticism, philosophy, systems theory, anthropology, and political theory.

But innovation also takes place within the boundaries of psychoanalysis, and Psychoanalysis in a New Key therefore also presents work that reformulates thought and practice without leaving the precincts of the field. Books in the series focus, for example, on the significance of personal values in psychoanalytic practice, on the complex interrelationship between the analyst's clinical work and personal life, on the consequences for the clinical situation when patient and analyst are from different cultures, and on the need for psychoanalysts to accept the degree to which they knowingly satisfy their own wishes during treatment hours, often to the patient's detriment. A full list of all titles in this series is available at: www.routledge.com/Psychoanalysis-in-a-New-Key-Book-Series/book-series/LEAPNKBS

Clara M. Thompson's Professional Evolution and Legacy

An American Psychoanalyst (1933-1958)

Ann D'Ercole

Routledge
Taylor & Francis Group

LONDON AND NEW YORK

Cover image: "Clara M. Thompson", Lotte Jacobi Collection. *University of New Hampshire*. Used with permission. © 2022 The University of New Hampshire.

First published 2023
by Routledge
4 Park Square, Milton Park, Abingdon, Oxon OX14 4RN

and by Routledge
605 Third Avenue, New York, NY 10158

Routledge is an imprint of the Taylor & Francis Group, an informa business

British Library Cataloguing-in-Publication Data
A catalogue record for this book is available from the British Library

Library of Congress Cataloging-in-Publication Data
Names: D'Ercole, Ann, author.
Title: Clara M. Thompson's professional evolution and legacy : an
    American psychoanalyst (1933–1958) / Ann D'Ercole, PhD, ABPP.
Description: Abingdon, Oxon ; New York, NY : Routledge, 2023. |
    Includes bibliographical references and index.
Identifiers: LCCN 2022016969 (print) | LCCN 2022016970 (ebook) |
    ISBN 9781032257525 (hardback) | ISBN 9781032257532
    (paperback) | ISBN 9781003284840 (ebook)
Subjects: LCSH: Thompson, Clara, 1893–1958. | Psychiatrists—United
    States—Biography. | Psychoanalysts—United States—Biography. |
    Psychoanalysis.
Classification: LCC RC438.6.T556 D47 2023 (print) | LCC
    RC438.6.T556 (ebook) | DDC 616.89/17092 [B]—dc23/
    eng/20220713
LC record available at https://lccn.loc.gov/2022016969
LC ebook record available at https://lccn.loc.gov/2022016970

Every effort has been made to contact copyright-holders. Please advise the publisher of any errors or omissions, and these will be corrected in subsequent editions.

ISBN: 978-1-032-25752-5 (hbk)
ISBN: 978-1-032-25753-2 (pbk)
ISBN: 978-1-003-28484-0 (ebk)

DOI: 10.4324/9781003284840

Typeset in Times New Roman
by Apex CoVantage, LLC

For Linda, Tony, David, Laura, Marci, Helen,
Andrew, Kaley, Frida, and Ryder.

Contents

Acknowledgments

There are so many individuals and institutions that made this book possible. Before thanking them, I want to say something about what it was like to do this work. Not only did I feel I got to know Clara Thompson; it felt as if she was my constant companion in the process. Conducting the research was absorbing and gratifying; the writing was more challenging. Writing is always difficult. Then, SARS COVID-19 descended on the world and sent me into isolation for what has now been close to two years. The virus brought dread, fear, and anxiety; I was privileged to isolate in Truro with my partner, Linda Brady. It was comforting having one of my sons and two of my grandchildren nearby, though at first our visits were limited to outdoors and wearing masks. This unprecedented situation allowed me to work on the project almost without interruption. Living through a pandemic was something I came to share with Clara Thompson.

This biography developed over years with many conversations with other psychoanalysts. I especially thank Dr. Edgar Levenson for his wise counsel and continuing support. His recollections and firsthand perspective have been an important influence. In 2018, I met Dr. Arnold Rachman, an expert on Sándor Ferenczi's work, and Ferenczi's patient, Elizabeth Severn. He was a muse who read drafts and provided valuable comments. He shared my excitement for the work. I am deeply grateful.

Support for the project came from many additional directions, including from my study group on interpersonal psychoanalysis (before SARS-COVID-19 sent us into isolation). It included Drs. Lynn Passy, Forbes Singer, Brenda Tepper, Catherine Baker-Pitts, and William Auerbach. My friends and colleagues, Anita Herron, Martin Devine, Barbara Suter, Jack Drescher, Judith Alpert, Nina Thomas, and Kenneth Eisold, read drafts and provided comments. Dr. Nellie Thompson, Curator, Archives & Special Collections, A.A. Brill Library/NYPSI, generously shared information and read a draft of a chapter. She introduced me to the work of Dr. Elizabeth Capelle. Capelle's dissertation traces important aspects of Clara Thompson's life. Her extensive research illuminated the role of Thompson's involvement with the Free Will Baptists and the critical feminist contributions made by Thompson. I have quoted widely from Capelle's work.

Christopher Busa, Peter Manso, and Anton Van Dereck Haunstrup helped to fill in details of life in Provincetown. Stephen Magliocco shared his architect's view of the memorials to Clara Thompson and Henry Major in the Provincetown Cemetery.

I thank Richard Herman, Director of Administration at William Alanson White (WAW), and Elizabeth Rodman, Administrative Manager, who made the archive at WAW available to me. Dr. Marylou Lionells, a former director of the William Alanson White Institute and co-editor of the *Handbook of Interpersonal Psychoanalysis*, graciously offered helpful comments and questions. Dr. Kenneth Eisold, esteemed author and current President of the Board at WAW, offered his support, read a chapter, and provided valuable comments. I thank and am indebted to Dr. Judith Dupont, for graciously responding to my questions, helping to clarify specific notations and some confusion Arnold Rachman and I had about the entries in the Clinical Diary of Sándor Ferenczi.

The New York University Postdoctoral Program in Psychotherapy and Psychoanalysis, my primary affiliation, is a generative community that fostered and encouraged this biography's necessity. Two past directors of the program are no doubt represented in these pages for their encouragement and foresight. Bernie Kalinkowitz, former New York University, Postdoctoral Program in Psychotherapy and Psychoanalysis (Postdoc) Director, was a patient of Clara Thompson's. Lewis Aron, a former Postdoc director, was sadly too ill to participate in the project, but he did encourage me to proceed. Lew was very interested in Clara Thompson's relationship to two of Ferenczi's patients, Izette de Forest and Elizabeth Severn, their complicated feelings toward each other. I hope I have begun to open up those feelings in the chapters.

I thank Elizabeth Capelle for reading several iterations of chapters and for her enormously helpful research into Thompson's life.

I am grateful to Donnel Stern, founder and editor of the Routledge series "Psychoanalysis in a New Key," for including this biography in the series and for his comments.

I thank Dr. Louis Rose, Executive Director, Sigmund Freud Archives, and Dr. Emanuel Garcia, Kurt Eissler's literary executor, for allowing the

1954 interview to be reprinted in the first volume in its entirety "without editorial emendations, typographical corrections, deletions, altered punctuation, or ellipses."

The Graduate Society of the Postdoctoral Program generously provided me with two Scholar's Grants supporting the project. They also gave me a forum for presenting this work early in its development.

I thank The Alan Mason Chesney Medical Archives of the Johns Hopkins Medical Institutions, specifically Marjorie W. Kehoe, Reference and Accessioning Archivist, who helped find the materials I requested. Likewise, Marisa Shaari at the DeWitt Wallace Institute for the History of Psychiatry & the Oskar Diethelm Library at Weill Cornell Medical College assisted in locating papers and correspondence. Librarians are critical to projects like this one. They reach out to other institutions and share generously. I thank them all. A special thank you to Dr. Rainer Funk, of the Literary Estate of Erich Fromm, Erich Fromm Institute Tubingen, for sending me an invaluable collection of Fromm/Thompson correspondence.

During the project, I sought out and received editorial assistance from Georgina Clutterbuck, Adrienne Hall, Anne Ranson, Kristopher Spring, Kim Bernstein, and my friend and colleague Jack Drescher. Each helped with different phases of the project and helped make the text flow smoothly, structuring it for publication.

My partner Linda Brady was an essential part of this journey. She encouraged, supported, and brought her perceptive clarity and questions to me as I structured this story.

My biographical history is a part of this book, too. Indeed, my parents, Rose Marion Iorio D'Ercole, and Raymond D'Ercole, would have delighted in the fact of this book. My children Laura, Tony, and David, and my daughters-in-law Marci and Helen have brought joy and sustenance, making a project like this possible. My daughter, Laura Mamo, a professor of sociology, lent her scholarly suggestions along the way. My granddaughters Kaley and Frida are excellent storytellers and writers. I hope they like this one. I appreciated Kaley's help with edits and our lunches at Terralucci. My grandson Andrew read and offered valuable comments early in writing. Thank you to my grandson Ryder for opening my eyes to what is now culturally relevant.

This book is also about all the psychoanalytic partners, patients, and analysts who undertake the treacherous and enormously gratifying journey of self-discovery. We are all pioneers.

Credits List

The author gratefully acknowledges the permission provided to republish the following materials:

- Analytic Observations during a course of a manic-depressive psychosis, Clara Thompson (ed.), *The Psychoanalytic Review*, 17(2). Republished with permission of Guilford Publications, Inc. © 1913; permission conveyed through Copyright Clearance Center, Inc.
- Audio material from Pembroke Center Oral History Collection, OH.1s.2013.002, Christine Dunlap Farnham Archive, Brown University Library.
- Clara Thompson, M.D. Interviewed by K. R. Eissler, M.D. June 4, 1952. Courtesy of Dr. Emanuel E. Garcia, the literary executor of the K.R. Eissler Estate, and Louis Rose, Executive Director, Sigmund Freud Archives. Sigmund Freud Papers: Interviews and Recollections, Set A, 1914–1998 (Box 122). Manuscripts Division, Library of Congress, Washington, DC. www.loc.gov/item/mss3999001575/
- "Concepts of the Self in Interpersonal Theory", Clara Thompson, *American Journal of Psychotherapy* 12(1), pp. 5–17. Reprinted with permission from the *American Journal of Psychotherapy*, (Copyright © 1958). American Psychiatric Association. All Rights Reserved.
- Documents and photographic material from the archive of the William Alanson White Institute, as provided by Richard Herman, Director of Administration at the Institute.
- Documents and correspondence from The Alan Mason Chesney Medical Archives, The Johns Hopkins University, The Johns Hopkins Hospital.

Timeline of Key Events

Move to NYC	1933
Reconnected with her mother	1933
Joins Zodiac Club with	
(Sullivan, Silverberg, Horney, others)	1933
Sullivan leaves New York for Baltimore	1939
Joins as faculty of New York Psychoanalytic Institute	1938
Meets Henry Majors at art exhibit (age 45)	1938
Purchase of Provincetown house	1938
Resigns New York Psychoanalytic Institute	1941
Letter to American Psychoanalytic Association:	
"A Crisis in Psychoanalytic Education."	1941
Establishment of American Association for the	
Advancement of Psychoanalysis and the	
American Institute of Psychoanalysis	1941–1943
Erich Fromm training privileges rejected	1943
William Alanson White Psychiatric Foundation	
reorganized its Washington School of Psychiatry	
with a New York Branch with Clara Thompson,	
Director	1943–1947
Henry Major illness and death	1947–1948
Death of Harry Stack Sullivan	1949
Erich Fromm moves to Mexico	1949
Death of Thompson's Mother	1952
Interview with Kurt Eissler	1952
Organizing the Academy of Psychoanalysis	1956
Malignant polyp detected	1956
Clara Thompson death 12/20 at age 65	1958

Introduction

Beginnings and Endings

As in Volume 1, *Clara M. Thompson's Early Years and Professional Awakening: An American Psychoanalyst (1893–1933)*, this narrative follows the practice of an oral history drawing on interviews, correspondence, and Clara Thompson's scholarly essays to allow the reader to discover whenever possible—Thompson in her own voice.

I have organized events in both volumes (1893–1933 and 1933–1958) chronologically, except for the first chapter in Volume 1, where I introduce Clara M. Thompson in her 1952 interview for the Freud Archive (Freud, S. 1952). The interview is essential to understanding the depth of Thompson's experience and the breadth of her perspective in the developing field of psychoanalysis. I refer to the interview throughout both volumes.

Clara M. Thompson's Professional Evolution and Legacy: An American Psychoanalyst (1933–1958) begins in New York City shortly after the death on May 22, 1933, of her beloved analyst, Sándor Ferenczi, at the age of 59. As she recounts in her 1952 interview, it was painful for them to say goodbye:

> He kept saying good-by to me in indirect ways, and I, several times I said, "But I'm coming to see you again this week," and then he'd say, "Oh, yes," and then again he would say good-by and he'd tell me what I should do in America, that I should carry on his ideas, and so forth. And I'd say, "but I'm not leaving Budapest, I'm coming to see you in a few days," and he'd say, "Oh, yes," but I think he must have felt that he would never see me again.

DOI: 10.4324/9781003284840-1

As she prepared to leave Budapest and move to New York, she said to her friend Izette de Forest (letter on February 26, 1933),[1]

> for the first time I really feel equal to New York and all its antagonisms, and having you and Alice there will certainly make it very pleasant . . . so we'll roll up our sleeves to go to it.
>
> (Brennan, 2009, p. 448)

At age 40, Thompson did roll up her sleeves and go to it. She felt supported by her friends and prepared to take up a new chapter of her life. Ferenczi's last request was for her to introduce his ideas to America. She also made a promise to her friend and colleague in New York, Harry Stack Sullivan, that she would analyze him as a means toward helping them both experience Ferenczi's therapeutic innovations. She kept her promise to Ferenczi, but she was selective. As she later said:

> I am a pupil of Ferenczi and for over ten years I have made use of some of his techniques in my psycho-analytic work. In the course of time I have discarded several of his ideas and confirmed the validity of others.
>
> (Thompson, 1943b, p. 64)

She also kept her promise to Sullivan, becoming his analyst in a treatment that lasted about three hundred hours. It ended abruptly when she tried to examine his pattern of financial overextension (Perry, 1982). (Perhaps she also tried to analyze his homosexuality.)

The most important aspect of Thompson's immersion in New York intellectual life, however, was her friendships, not only with Sullivan but with two other analysts, Karen Horney and Erich Fromm. All four lived near one another, gathering frequently for meetings that Thompson characterized as "scientific social": a mix of peer supervision, study group, and forum for discussion about their own psychoanalytic work as well as current understandings of the unconscious, transference, countertransference, the role of the analyst, and the contributions of culture, empathy and society. The quartet soon expanded to include other psychoanalysts and social scientists. During the early years, the core group that met regularly and was officially named by Sullivan as the Zodiac Club.

Thompson and Horney in particular shared a feminist critique of Freud's developmental theories. Thompson's views were more controversial than those of Horney. She challenged psychoanalysts to think in terms of equality—of the similarties between women and men, rather than the biological differences. While she stayed within a binary frame, she held firmly to cultural considerations:

> Sexual difference is an obvious difference, and obvious differences are especially convenient marks of derogation in any competitive situation in which one group aims to get power over the other.
>
> (Thompson, 1943, p. 124)

Women, she argued are trapped between two opposing ideas: self-fulfillment; service to others. She herself had experienced that tension when she struggled to resolve the intellectual conflicts between the teachings of her religious community and her Pembroke/Brown professors. Unlike Horney, she did not subscribe to the argument that women had special qualities resulting from bodily experiences, such as menstruation, pregnancy, and childbirth. Instead Thompson underscored society's discrepant messages and conflicting expectations for women. In short, she was a 20th century woman whose feminism was ahead of its time.

During this intellectually fertile period, Clara Thompson chose to undergo a third psychoanalytic treatment, with Erich Fromm. While she still missed Ferenczi, she chose Fromm because she believed that he would understand an aspect of her personality that Ferenczi had overlooked: She used her aggression to manipulate others.

Fromm's focus on loneliness and alienation would have been appealing to her. As she said, "[A]ccording to Fromm, man is constantly tempted, to go back to some form of relatedness to his fellows, even at the price of giving up some of his individuality" (Thompson, 1979, p. 196). Overall, her work with Fromm left her feeling stronger, more resilient, "less a frightened child in a hostile world" as she later wrote in her letter to Fromm, April 2, 1956 (courtesy of Dr. Ranier Funk, the Erich Fromm Archive, Tubingen). One could say with Ferenczi she found her voice, and with Fromm she learned how to use it, particularly in her emerging presence in the psychoanalytic community.[2]

At Horney's urging, she joined the New York Psychoanalytic Society. That affiliation ended, however, when Horney received a demotion that prompted not just her and Thompson but four other faculty members and fourteen students to leave the Society in protest (Thompson, 2017). The group then formed the Advancement of Psychoanalysis and the American Institute for Psychoanalysis. A power struggle soon ensued there, too, one in which Horney was instrumental in excluding Erich Fromm from the status of training analyst. A repeat in some ways of what happened to her at New York Psychoanalytic.

In 1943, Thompson, Sullivan, Fromm, and others broke with Horney and formed the Washington School of Psychiatry. By some accounts the reference to "psychiatry" in the school's name led the American Psychoanalytic to reject the Washington school as not psychoanalysis. Thompson rejoined the Washington-Baltimore Society and was reapproved as a member of the American Psyhcoanalytic. But then the American established a new rule that allowed only one training institute in a city. The members of the Washington-Baltimore Society were told they "[s]hould apply for recognition as a separate institute" (Thompson, 2017, p. 22). In a series of lost paperwork, and requests for new information, another new rule was instituted, and membership denied. The sequence of these events and ensuing dramas are complicated and difficult to follow. I have chosen to stay close to Thompson's descriptions when possible.

In 1946, the Washington-Baltimore Society in New York became The William Alanson White Institute, with Clara Thompson installed as Executive Director. In 1951, the name was changed to William Alanson White Institute of Psychiatry, Psychoanalysis and Psychology, with Thompson remaining as Director.

Even as Thompson was building a successful professional life, a significant change was happening in her personal life. In 1938, she met and fell in love with Henry Major, a Hungarian artist. She purchased a house in Provincetown, MA, where she and Major lived in the summers. In the winter, Major lived with his wife Elizabeth Alexander. Thompson and Major's unconventional life in Provincetown was a good fit with local fisherman, artists, intellectuals, and rebels. Major was an artist of international renown. He worked for the Hearst Paper as a caricaturist and covered the Lindbergh kidnapping trial rendering drawings of the events. Their relationship lasted until his death in 1948.

Thompson's letters to Ralph Crowley, portray Provincetown as a place of respite and love. The correspondence describes her busy social life and shows her long-distance attention attend to the administrative demands of the institute.

Thompson as Intellectual

I have drawn from Thompson's essays in order to both bring her voice into the narrative and, add her substantial intellectual contributions to the discussion. She spent her career building what Lionells (1995) called "a series of bridges between the sociopolitical concerns of Fromm and the innovations of Sullivan" in clinical technique (p. 63) and incorporating the leading-edge psychiatry of Adolf Meyer with the creative psychoanalytic innovations of Ferenczi, Sullivan, Horney, and Fromm.

Thompson's contributions to the psychology of women were substantial and are still relevant. Our challenge is to understand her pioneering contributions within the context of her time. With little fanfare or acknowledgment, mainstream psychoanalysis has absorbed Thompson's clinical concepts. Thompson (1979) used Fromm's observations to say, "society not only curbs some needs, but also creates new needs" (p. 195).[3] She embraced Sullivan's interest in culture and his focus on, "what goes on between people, especially in the areas of interaction, which seemed to create difficulties in living" (p. 199). In her essay, "Dutiful Child: Resistance"[4] (1931), she introduced the concept of compliance as a form of resistance not only in childhood development but in clinical treatment. Her case material can often read as autobiography in disguise.

In her (1938a) ground-breaking essay, she described a changing field of clinical practice. "Notes on the Psychoanalytic Significance of the Choice of Analyst" was published in Sullivan's new journal, *Psychiatry*. It was written five years after the death of Ferenczi. Thompson introduces the concept of reciprocity in the analytic encounter and shifts the focus from trying to understand the mind of the analysand, to discovering the continuous dynamic relationship between the analyst and analysand. She was, in effect, articulating a new interpretation of the psychoanalytic process. This is something she no doubt acquired first-hand in her work with Ferenczi.

Thompson's legacy also includes her role as historian. *Psychoanalysis: Evolution and Development* (1950) a collection of lectures Thompson had given over the decades at various schools and institutes, provides a more-or-less definitive history of the period in 1920s Europe when Otto Rank, Sándor Ferenczi and Wilhelm Reich were considered rebels.

In 1955, at a meeting of the Harry Stack Sullivan Society, Thompson chronicled The History of the William Alanson White Institute (Published in 2017). In that essay, she recounts the divisiveness, disruptions, and triumphs she encountered in American psychoanalytic training organizations and her role in the process of their development.

Characteristic of Thompson, she can slide past the parts that would identify her significance,[5] or resort to humor "—that's my fate, to be the first president of something" (Thompson, 2017, p. 14).

In her essays, Thompson used the terms[6] interpersonal relations, interpersonal theory, interpersonal process, and interpersonal forces in describing her understanding of human behavior and the clinical psychoanalytic method. In 1964, Maurice Green organized her articles and unpublished papers into *Interpersonal Psychoanalysis: The Selected Papers of Clara Mabel Thompson* a title that speaks unambiguously to her theorizing and clinical acumen. By choosing the title *Interpersonal Psychoanalysis*, Green confirms her leadership in the interpersonal psychoanalytic tradition.

Gone Missing

Thompson encouraged her students to find their own analytic voice rather than copying hers—an admirable approach, perhaps, but one that wound up obscuring her contributions. Despite her many accomplishments, Clara Thompson was quickly erased from our psychoanalytic history. As Edgar Levenson remarked, "[O]nce she was dead, she was gone" (personal communication).

Today, Thompson's essays stand as evidence of her contribution to the field as do the testimonials of her students, analysands, and colleagues—the beneficiaries of her work as a clinical supervisor, psychoanalyst, and theoretician. And they are not alone: We are all beneficiaries of Thompson's contributions. She brought a unique emotional immediacy to her therapeutic work—respect for, and openness to, the analytic encounter that several generations of interpersonalists have embraced.

As I wrote in ending the first volume of this biography, I hope in telling Clara Mabel Thompson's story I have added to what we know, increased its accuracy, and, in the tradition of an oral history, encouraged others to keep her story alive. I think of this story as a conversation that has not ended.

Notes

1 The date of this letter confusingly precedes Ferenczi's death.
2 See Frosch (1991) for a good description of the New York psychoanalytic wars.
3 This essay was written in 1956, appeared in *Interpersonal Psychoanalysis; The Selected Papers of Clara Thompson* (1964). Ed. by M. R. Green. New York: Basic Books. It was reprinted in 1979 in *Contemporary Psychoanalysis*, Vol. 15, No 2.
4 Read before the Washington-Baltimore Psychoanalytic Society, November 15, 1930. Published in *Interpersonal Psychoanalysis; The Selected Papers of Clara Thompson* (1964). Ed. by M. R. Green. New York: Basic Books.
5 She was in Baltimore and part of those early conversations, when the Washington-Baltimore Psychoanalytic Society was established, she became its first president.
6 "Interpersonal relations" (1978, p. 492, 1979, p. 196, 1988, p. 194, 2017, p. 8), "interpersonal theory" (2017, p. 11), "interpersonal process" (1978, p. 496), and "interpersonal forces" (1978, p. 50). The 1978 paper first appeared in *The Contributions of Harry Stack Sullivan* (1952). Ed. by P. Mullahy. New York: Hermitage Press. The 1979 paper was first written in 1956, this essay appeared in *Interpersonal Psychoanalysis; The Selected Papers of Clara Thompson* (1964). Ed. by M. R. Green. New York: Basic Books.

References

Brennan, B. W. (2009). Ferenczi's forgotten messenger: The life and work of Izette de Forest. *American Imago*, *66*(4), 427–455.

Freud, S. (1952). Interview with Clara Thompson (K. R. Eissler, Interviewer). Manuscript/mixed material. Sigmund Freud Papers: Interviews and Recollections, Set A, 1914–1998 (Box 122). Manuscripts Division, Library of Congress, Washington, DC. www.loc.gov/item/mss3999001575/

Frosch, J. (1991). The New York psychoanalytic civil war. *Journal of the American Psychoanalytic Association*, *39*(4), 1037–1064.

Green, M. R. (Ed.). (1964). *Interpersonal psychoanalysis: The selected papers of Clara M. Thompson*. New York: Basic Books.

Lionells, M. (1995). *Interpersonal-Relational Psychoanalysis: an Introduction and Overview of Contemporary Implications and Applications International Forum of Psychoanalysis*, *4*(4), 223–230.

Lionells, M. (1996). Clara M. Thompson (1893–1958), Some effects of the derogatory attitude toward female sexuality (Introduction by Marylou Lionells). In D. B. Stern, C. H. Mann, S. Kantor, & G. Schlesginger (Eds.), *Pioneers of Interpersonal Psychoanalysis* (pp. 61–72). Hillsdale, NJ: The Analytic Press.

Perry, H. S. (1982). *Psychiatrist of America, the life of Harry Stack Sullivan.* Cambridge, MA and London: Belknap Press of Harvard University Press.

Thompson, C. (1931). Dutiful child resistance. *Psychoanalytic Review, 18,* 426–434.

Thompson, C. (1943a). "Penis Envy" in Women, *Psychiatry, 6*(2), 123–125, DOI: 10.1080/00332747.1943.11022443

Thompson, C. (1943b). The therapeutic technique of Sándor Ferenczi: A comment. *International Journal of Psychoanalysis, 24,* 64–66.

Thompson, C. (1978) Sullivan and psychoanalysis. *Contemporary Psychoanalysis, 14*(4), 488–501.

Thompson, C. (1979). Sullivan and Fromm. *Contemporary Psychoanalysis, 15,* 195–200.

Thompson, C. (1988). Sándor Ferenczi, 1873–1933. *Contemporary Psychoanalysis, 24,* 182–195.

Thompson, C. (2017). The history of the William Alanson White Institute. *Contemporary Psychoanalysis, 53*(1), 7–28.

Chapter 1

Thompson, Sullivan, Fromm, and Horney

Clara Thompson's professional evolution began at Johns Hopkins School of Medicine when she chose psychiatry as her field of specialization. However, it is in 1933, with her move to New York that she turned the full force of her ambition toward her professional life. She could have returned to Baltimore but as Erich Fromm recalled, she relocated to New York to "[g]et away from Baltimore" (Fromm, letter to Ralph Crowley dated April 5, 1968, courtesy of Oskar Diethelm Library, Ralph Crowley Papers). She needed to distance herself from her conflicts with Adolf Meyer and the Phipps Clinic. She considered of those years at the clinic in Baltimore as the most challenging and emotionally taxing years of her life.

In this second volume of Clara Thompson's biography, we meet her at age 40, in New York City. It is 1933; Sándor Ferenczi's death that year had been difficult for her to accept. During her last visits with him, he would say "goodbye" while she maintained "I'll see you tomorrow."[1] Her analysis from 1927 to 1933 had left her feeling less inhibited, more open, and less lonely. She now felt stronger but missed Ferenczi and longed to continue her personal analytic work. In 1934, she began a third analysis with Erich Fromm (Funk, 2000, p. 106). With Fromm's help, she overcame, as she described it, feeling like "a frightened child in a hostile world" (Thompson, letter to Fromm, April 2, 1956, courtesy of Dr. Ranier Funk, the Erich Fromm Archive, Tubingen).

Her move to 151 East 83rd Street on the upper east side of New York situated her near friends, particularly her close friend, Harry Stack Sullivan, and his partner James (Jimmie) Inscoe, who lived on East 64th Street. By then Jimmie was about 21 and a close friend as well. In 1934, when Erich Fromm initially moved to New York, he resided for a short time with

DOI: 10.4324/9781003284840-2

Sullivan and Inscoe. He then moved to East 66th Street before relocating to be near the new home of the Institute for Social Research at Columbia University (Funk, 2000). Karen Horney initially moved to the residential Surrey Hotel, at 20 East 76th Street just off Madison Avenue.

In New York, Clara Thompson was surrounded by a group of distinguished intellectuals and close friends. On Sundays, the crowd assembled at Clara Thompson's home for spirited discussions and parties. They also met weekly at Karen Horney's hotel apartment to eat, drink, and share psychoanalytic viewpoints. Thompson and Horney were friends who shared similar views about women in society and had in common, critiques of Freud's developmental theories. The group included Columbia University's leading anthropologists Margaret Mead and Ruth Benedict, among other legends; John Dollard, an American psychologist and social scientist known for his studies on race relations and early theories on frustration and aggression; Harold Lasswell, a University of Chicago graduate and Yale University professor in law, known for his contributions to understanding personality, social structure, and culture in political phenomena; Abram Kardiner, a psychiatrist interested in the study of culture and the traumatic effects of war; William Silverberg, a Washington-Baltimore psychoanalytic training program graduate and founder of the Academy of Psychoanalysis. Sullivan was busy with his lecture series traveling back and forth along the Washington-Baltimore-New York-Chicago route. His biographer Perry (1982) maintains, he rarely lost sight of his goal "—to make life meaningful and productive for more and more people" (p. 261). That goal was shared by Thompson, Fromm, and Horney.

Clara Thompson was a perennial intellectual bridge builder. She connected the therapeutic discoveries she made with Ferenczi with her prior psychiatric training under Adolf Meyer at Johns Hopkins as she linked ideas arising in discussions with Harry Stack Sullivan and other colleagues from the Washington-Baltimore area. Sullivan's work had shown that even in disturbed populations, individuals were capable of attachment and like Ferenczi's work he too proved, patients were sensitive to the analyst's personality. Clara Thompson's interest was drawn to the therapeutic encounter itself as demonstrated by her 1938 essay, *Notes on the Psychoanalytic Significance of the Choice of Analyst*. Her essay influenced the transformation of the practice of psychoanalysis in America, bringing in a two-person view of psychoanalytic treatment.

Professional Evolution: The influence of Sullivan, Horney, and Fromm

Clara Thompson's professional development and contributions were indelibly shaped by her connections with Harry Stack Sullivan, Karen Horney, Erich Fromm, and a wide range of intellectuals across various fields. Elizabeth Capelle (1998) offers a fitting description for Thompson, Sullivan, Horney, and Fromm as a "diverse quartet" (p. 85). They worked, played, and listened to one another as they became more established professionally. One of the many benefits of their overlapping friendships was the creation of a synergy of influences in their professional development. There were meetings, parties, patients, and students mixed with institutional politics and vital intimate relationships. As friends, they would dine together, go to the theater, and visit art museums and exhibitions. They agreed on the importance of the role of sociocultural context in the shaping of personality. They were friends, colleagues, and for a time, analysts and analysands. In the case of Horney and Fromm, they had a long-standing romantic relationship. Overall, their attachment to one another was supportive, competitive, and enlivening.

Friends: Strong Connections

Thompson and Horney met at Baden-Baden. They became better acquainted when Horney visited the Washington-Baltimore Psychoanalytic Society for a meeting of the American Psychoanalytic Association where Thompson and Sullivan were in attendance. In 1932, Horney had left Berlin for Chicago at the invitation of Franz Alexander, a Hungarian American psychoanalyst and first graduate of the Berlin Psychoanalytic Institute. Alexander invited her to be his "assistant" in setting up a psychoanalytic institute at the university after Helen Deutsch declined the position (Rubins, 1978, pp. 127–128). In Chicago, Horney met Sullivan and became friends with the psychiatrist Lionel Blitsten, who had attended Horney's course in Berlin (Rubins, 1978, p. 168). She became friends with Dorothy Blitsten, a psychoanalyst and sociologist who was married to Lionel, the psychiatrist Ralph Crowley, the anthropologist, Edward Sapir, and the sociologist Harold Lasswell; all friends of Sullivan's and now of Horney's at the University of Chicago. Filling in the Chicago circle was Erich Fromm, who was a guest lecturer at the Institute. This is where

Horney wrote her first papers in English on women. Moulton (1975) suggests that Horney's lack of a personal bond with Freud separated her from women who had worked closely with him, and the distance freed her to make her differences from him clearer during the years of her associations with Thompson, Sullivan, and Fromm. As Horney's two-year contract with the Chicago Institute ended, her relationship with Alexander became strained. In 1934, she made the decision to leave Chicago. She sold her car and used the money to finance her move to New York. At the age of 50, New York became another start following her immigration from Berlin (Rubin, 1978). She left her daughters in Chicago and for the first time was living alone. In New York, Horney began to focus on a wider philosophy of treatment based on basic human needs.

Thompson and Sullivan were more than best friends; they had become family. They met in Baltimore in 1923 when Thompson was a psychiatric resident and Sullivan was working as a veterans' liaison officer at St. Elizabeth's Hospital, Washington, DC. They immediately took to each other. Perry (1982) notes that over the years, they were loyal, supportive friends who could privately "criticize each other" (p. 201). Thompson like Horney knew Sullivan's friends from Chicago. She became close to his partner, James Inscoe beginning in Baltimore when they frequently dined together. Sullivan's relationship with Inscoe lasted decades. Following Sullivan's death, Thompson and Jimmie remained friends.

When Erich Fromm moved to New York, he was still recovering from a bout of tuberculosis suffered in the summer of 1931 (Funk, 2019). Over the next several years of his life, he struggled with the sequalae of the illness. He was no longer living with his wife Frieda Fromm-Reichmann, though his divorce was not official. Thompson and he had likely met at Baden-Baden in 1932, the Twelfth International Psycho-Analytical Congress at Wiesbaden, where Ferenczi gave his groundbreaking paper, *Confusion of Tongues*. In the years that followed, Fromm taught at the New School for Social Research, while Karen Horney taught at the New York Psychoanalytic Institute and after her urging, Clara Thompson too taught at New York Psychoanalytic, where she was a training analyst.

Horney and Fromm's friendship began in Berlin, years before they moved to New York. In 1934, their friendship morphed into a romantic relationship (Friedman, 2013). Horney hoped they would marry after his divorce, but by the time his marriage to Frieda Fromm-Reichman officially ended in 1940, their relationship too was over. Neither Fromm nor Horney was monogamous; Friedman (2013) explains that Horney had a reputation of having affairs with younger men who were her analysands or supervisees. Fromm's relationship with Katherine Dunham, an American dancer, seems to have caused Horney the most anguish, so much that when she split with him, she insisted his friend Ernst Schachtel stop seeing Fromm. When he did not, she broke with him as well (Funk, 2000, p. 117). Further complicating Fromm and Horney's relationship, in 1937, Horney referred her daughter Marianne, a psychiatric resident at New York's Payne-Whitney Clinic, to Fromm for her training analysis. Fromm and Horney were competitive and ambitious. To use Fromm's language, Horney wanted a partner, a "magic helper"; Fromm wanted his freedom (Friedman, 2013, p. 82). Thompson explains that Fromm was a critic of Western culture, his views challenged humanity:

> He (sic) must learn to think, He becomes aware of his powerlessness in a cosmic setting: he becomes conscious that he must die; he feels more alone. On the other hand, he has become more free and can develop his powers more and more, resulting in greater mastery over nature. His own creations, machines and the like, have separated him more and more from his earlier contacts with nature. Loneliness and a feeling of alienation are becoming his fate in the Western culture. According to Fromm, man is constantly tempted, therefore, to go back to some form of relatedness to his fellows, even at the price of giving up some of his individuality.
>
> (Thompson, 1979, p. 195)[2]

Erich Fromm and Harry Stack Sullivan shared many similar world views and enjoyed learning from one another as they joined with other intellectuals from the culture-and-personality movement. Clara Thompson describes them in her paper, *Sullivan and Fromm* (1979), she says,

> About 1934, Sullivan and Fromm met for the first time, and for several years thereafter there was a working collaboration between them at the Washington School of Psychiatry and the William Alanson White Institute. They held certain concepts in common, but each preserved his own particular approach to the problems. The work of

each supplements the other, and their <u>basic assumptions</u> about human beings are similar. The chief area which they share in common is the interest in the impact of cultural pressures on <u>personality develop-ment</u>. The chief area of difference is in theories about <u>the self</u>.

(p. 195)

She continues,

> The contributions of Sullivan and Fromm have come to be called the "cultural school," because of the great emphasis of both on the interpersonal factors in personality formation and personal difficul-ties and the relative lack of emphasis on the more biologic drives as dynamic factors.

(p. 200)

Thompson could have enriched this paper by locating herself in the nar-rative, pointing her readers to the fact that she was a contributor to the "cultural school" of psychoanalysis. But it would have been bold and out of character for her to situate herself alongside these men. In the same way, she did not place herself inside her 1952 discussion of *Sullivan and Psy-choanalysis* (1978). Her early foundational experiences left her with a lin-gering humility that did not allow her to be self-promoting. Also, given the expansive personalities of these two men, she would have needed sharp elbows for her to assume the equal stature she deserved.

During this period, Fromm was concerned with the war in Europe. He regularly sent money to his family and friends and helped arrange for their escape from the Nazis. In 1939, at the Frankfurt Institute located at Colum-bia University, a salary dispute took place between Fromm, Horkheimer, and Pollock. They settled the dispute for the sum of twenty thousand dol-lars (Wheatland, 2009, p. 83) which gave Fromm a small financial cushion to augment his private practice.

Sullivan's homosexuality was an essential aspect of his life. Blechner (2005) suggests that Sullivan was "a pathbreaker in dealing with many of today's issues of gay civil rights" (p. 1). However, gay pride was decades away from Sullivan. There were no openly gay psychiatrists in the early 20th century.[3] For Sullivan, such a pronouncement would have resulted in being ostracized, arrested, or worse.

Perhaps, part of Sullivan's living beyond his financial means, incurring substantial debts and bankruptcy, was associated with his lingering sense of shame and outsider status. Drescher (2017) says of Sullivan,

> He lived at a time when homosexuality was illegal in all 50 states and public exposure could potentially lead to loss of one's medical license, one's academic position, and loss of referrals. Even today, it is not entirely clear to me how Sullivan, whose homosexuality seemed to be an open secret, got a get-out-of-jail-free pass.
>
> (p. 32)

Thompson and Sullivan enjoyed what appears to be a devoted attachment to one another and yet curiously their attitudes toward homosexuality were less than positive; more as Drescher might say, "[D]on't ask don't tell" than "out and proud." Their defensive styles were not dissimilar. Both relied on dissociative processes that were perhaps an adaptation to a biased culture. Sullivan viewed dissociative operations as ubiquitous; they made life more manageable (Drescher, 2017).

During these early years in New York, Clara Thompson was still feeling the effects of Ferenczi's death. It must have been a comfort to her that her housekeeper Lillie Fisher relocated with her to New York together with Harry Stack and Jimmie living nearby. In 1934, she reconciled with her mother after a nearly two-decade estrangement. She told her friend Ilona Vass (Shapiro, 1993, p. 168) that she was looking forward to spending part of her vacation with her mother. Then, at the age of 45, her romantic life blossomed, Clara Thompson fell in love with the artist Henry Major.

Up till now, Thompson's love life did not consist of any long-term relationship. It is Thompson's friend the psychoanalyst Zeborah Schachtel (personal communication) who affirmed that Thompson was bisexual, lending some support to Shapiro's (1993) statement that Thompson "like many great women of her generation . . . kept her insecurities, longings, and need for comfort from other women closeted as well while working for a day when that would be unnecessary" (p. 171). We must live with the historical uncertainty of these intimate details of Thompson's life. We do know that it was Henry Major with whom she established a long-term relationship.

During this period, Karen Horney published the *Neurotic Personality of Our Time* (1937); Fromm published, *Escape from Freedom* in 1941;

Thompson published, *Psychoanalysis: Evolution and Development* in 1950. Sullivan, a prolific writer, gave a series of lectures; most were recorded and preserved. *Conceptions of Modern Psychiatry*, published as an entire issue of the journal *Psychiatry* in 1945 by William Alanson White Psychiatric Foundation. These successes also led to rivalries.

Thompson and Horney each became organizational leaders. As a colleague who knew them both commented,

> even though both had needs for leadership, domination and prestige, Karen was more like 'a brunnhilde . . . in her carriage, dignity, forcefulness, and charisma. . . . Clara was more tender, encouraging and emotionally involved.
>
> (Rubins, 1978, p. 188)

In a sexist society, the personality characteristics deemed acceptable for women in authority remain controversial and problematic (Silver, 1996). Perhaps, Thompson's less assertive style found more acceptance though she seems to have permitted the men to receive credit, marginalizing her accomplishments.

Sullivan ultimately moved back to Baltimore but continued to stay involved with the group. The romantic relationship between Horney and Fromm ended with resentments. Clara Thompson and Sullivan remained close throughout life despite Sullivan's abrupt termination of treatment. In her treatment of him, she had tried to intervene in his financial decisions; Sullivan abruptly ended the analysis after about 300 hours between December 1934 to February 1936.[4] Perry (1982) says that Thompson, "tried to discourage him from extensive remodeling and elaborate plans for decoration, predicting that he would go into bankruptcy." And that Sullivan said, he "could not work with someone who had such 'bourgeois values'" (p. 214).

Perry (1982) believed that Sullivan, "yearned to be rich so he could do all kinds of things for people in need" (p. 213). As Thompson predicted, Sullivan did go into bankruptcy, an embarrassment he felt for the rest of his life. On February 27, 1936, Thompson wrote to her friend, Izette de Forest about the termination of her analytic work with Sullivan:

> H. S. S. has left me. His final dream was that he and a favorite woman patient (who left him in order to be able to meet him socially) were

sitting side by side in a very affectionate manner. He wouldn't give any of his associations to this—in fact in the past two months he has had many thoughts which he has refused to mention because then I might think the analysis was getting somewhere and he wants me to stop. For the past few weeks he has talked frequently of keeping on a few more weeks to save my self-esteem. He finally stopped because I asked him why be so altruistic. He is murderously angry with me, still a lot of ideas have been passed to him—all of them officially rejected with jeers but who knows what he's been thinking about them. Anyway as he left he acted very friendly and said he thought we ought to break a bottle of wine over this. I said I thought we'd better let it ride for a while. I wish I knew what has really happened, whether anyone else could have done better with him, whether my achieving my own emancipation from him perhaps led me to be too sadistic in pointing out things, who knows.

(Brennan, 2009, p. 448)

Thompson's letter to de Forest supports the idea that she might have been too hard on him. Her essay *The Interpersonal Approach to the Clinical Problems of Masochism* (1959a) may also be relevant to her analytic work with Sullivan. There she discusses some of the problems encountered when conducting therapy with a particularly difficult personality. The person wants to change she argues, but not enough—not enough to give up their protective character defenses designed to cope with anxiety.

The Zodiac Club

In Baltimore, Clara Thompson, William Silverberg, and Harry Stack Sullivan had a tradition of meeting in a speakeasy over drinks and dinner to discuss patients. They called themselves the Miracle Club because they concluded that their discussions led to the patient's improvement (Perry, 1982, p. 354).

In New York, Thompson, Sullivan, Horney, and Silverberg met on Mondays for dinner, drinks, and lively conversation. Sullivan named their gathering the Zodiac Club.

The Zodiac Club had what Thompson called a "scientific social," agenda, a combination of peer supervision, study group, and socialization (Thompson, 2017). They were in effect a brain trust of psychoanalysts.

Sullivan named each participant after an animal, thought to reflect their personalities: Sullivan a horse, Thompson a puma, Silverberg a gazelle, Shipley an okapi, Jimmie (Harry's partner) a seahorse, and Horney a water buffalo (Rubins, 1978). Sullivan used the symbol of a horse his entire life (Chapman, 1976). He was fond of drawing two horse heads—enclosed in a circle, one looking up, the other down—an emblem that was partially derived from an ancient Chinese symbol for eternal life. It appeared on the title pages of his posthumously published books, and he used it in various ways during his life. There are many interpretations of the Horse symbol as Perry describes on p. 343.

The Zodiac Group expanded over time to include various anthropologists, the photographer Margaret Bourke-White, and other individuals from the arts. Erich Fromm dropped in occasionally but was not a regular member.

We don't know whether Sullivan was familiar with the original Zodiac Club, a secret dining society that met from 1868 until 1928 (Oteri, 2013). Membership was limited to 12 at any one time because each member was assigned a zodiacal sign unrelated to their birth sign. The 12 were highly wealthy men who met for lavish dinners in New York on the last Saturday of every month. By contrast, the psychoanalytic Zodiac Club was not limited to men or wealth. It initially met weekly in speakeasies, during prohibition, and then in the homes of members.

Stories

The writer Harry Biele's story reveals a playfulness (with suggestive undertones) in Thompson and Sullivan's relationship.

> When at a party, Clara [Thompson] wearing a dress covered with dry sequins asks HSS [Harry Stack Sullivan] how he liked it. He walked over to her and shut his eyes, running his hands along the dress like a blind man . . . [He said] "it's like moving your hand against millions of nipples at the speed of light."
>
> (Wake, 2011, p. 146)

We need to reevaluate Thompson and Sullivan's connection in light of the fact that Sullivan was a gay man. As a man he could get away with this type of heteronormative behavior, which could be understood as a kind of playful ruse that allowed him (and perhaps her) to get away with their otherwise non-normative behavior(s). This might also answer Drescher's (2017) question of how did Sullivan, a gay psychiatrist in the middle of the 20th century, manage to come by a "get out of jail free pass" (p. 32) in terms of his public sexual identity. Perhaps also in humor, Sullivan gave a photo of himself wearing the US Medical Corps uniform, formally inscribed, to "Dr. Clara Thompson." They clearly enjoyed different aspects of themselves.

Perry (1982) recalling the man whose marriage proposal Thompson turned down in college curiously suggests,

> Two officers in Medical Corps had rejected Clara Thompson in different ways. The first had rejected her right to intellectual achievement; the other had steadfastly accorded her that right, but he had denied her the love of a man for a woman.
>
> (p. 214)

Perry's unrequited love story imposes a heteronormative model onto Thompson and Sullivan's relationship, rather than seeing their closeness as what we might think of as a chosen kinship connection.

Another interesting story is told by Clifford Read[5] in an unpublished manuscript, dated 1/27 titled "Harry Stack Sullivan: A Remembrance." Read explains that his memories of Sullivan are "filtered through conversations about Sullivan with Clara Thompson and my close friend Ralph Crowley." Read, who worked at a "Socialist radio station," met Sullivan when Sullivan spoke on a broadcast about the Scottsboro boys accused of rape and facing death in Alabama. He was impressed with Sullivan's warmth and confidence. Read later went to see Sullivan about his brother Billy who was "sometimes locked in catatonia and at others, trying to beat up attendants or patients. A very disturbed patient" (p. 5). Sullivan thought Billy's prognosis was poor. Over time, Sullivan and Read became friends. Read describes one of their last nights out alone when during a dinner Sullivan described the pleasures of Turkish baths. After dinner, Sullivan asked him if he would like to go to a Turkish bath with him. Read was startled and unwilling, and as they rode in a taxi in silence Sullivan sensed his hesitation and said, "[W]hatever happened at the Turkish bath would be confusing and complicating for him." He withdrew his invitation. A few weeks later they were to have dinner, but Sullivan forgot, blaming Jimmie for not reminding him of the date. Then Read calls Sullivan and tells him he had decided to "try analysis myself." Sullivan responds with enthusiasm saying he will introduce him to a couple of possible analysts.

> A patient of his had written a play for the radical Theater Union . . . why didn't we all go to the opening? We must wear black ties, Dr. Sullivan decided. Dressing for the Theater Union that prided itself on being revolutionary seemed to me the wrong ideas and I explained that this would be an open collar occasion. Nonsense, we were taking Dr. Clara Thompson and we couldn't dress like peasants. So four of us sat in formal dress in an audience of sweaters and jeans, not as working class as the producers hoped, but certainly belligerently against convention and capitalism.
>
> (Read, p. 22)

After the play they went to a speakeasy. "Harry Stack said we all needed alcohol to replace adrenalin. The psychiatrists began to talk of the play and projection, and I asked what the work meant." Sullivan explained "projection was a device for putting on others responsibility for feelings of your own. (Harry Stack smiled and gestured as he explained.) Thus, he said, he often saw those around him as grim and threatening while Clara saw them as benign and friendly" (p. 23).

As they drank, Read looked at the three psychiatrists and tried to decide which one he might choose as his analyst. Sullivan had told him he would only work with him

> if he felt that he alone could help. If I chose Dr. Silverberg, I would probably turn out in the way that Harry Stack felt was right for me. If I chose Dr. Thompson—well, he did not know how I would shape up.
>
> (p. 23)

Read felt there was much warmth in Sullivan but that there was also something demanding. He thought if he worked with him, "I would wind up being interested only in men." Silverberg was interested in music and Read was tone deaf. He found Thompson to be "perceptive and friendly, I felt comfortable with her. So I chose her and began many years on the couch, five times a week at five dollars an hour." "Goodness," my mother said, "[S]he must be getting rich. Mother wanted to help, though, and wrote Dr. Thompson offering to answer any questions about my childhood."

Read's mother was "miffed" when Clara answered, suggesting she tell Read anything she felt important. (p. 23)

The psychoanalyst Joseph Lichtenberg[6] shared a story he heard from Lewis Hill about Thompson.

> I never had direct contact with Clara Thompson, but my mentor, Lewis Hill, was at Sheppard Pratt and Clara Thompson was his analyst. Lewis was the most brilliant therapist I've ever known. He went to Budapest for a summer to be analyzed by Ferenczi. When Lewis came back from there, he went into analysis with Clara Thompson. I will tell you one story about Clara Thompson that he told me. Lewis is on the couch, and he is pausing, fumbling around. She says, "What are you thinking?" "I'm looking at your legs." And she said, "They are ugly?" And he said, "Yes," and she said, "Any idea of what I can do about it?" That's how she was.

Toward a New Understanding of the Psychoanalytic Encounter

Thompson's work with Ferenczi had changed her along with her understanding of psychotherapeutic work. Certain themes crystalized. She had experienced first-hand, what we today might call a sharing of subjectivities. They explored their intersubjective worlds sharing their conscious and unconscious thoughts. This is the most challenging work even for analysts today. This turn toward the influence of relationships on both psychological development and in clinical work began with Ferenczi (Thompson, 1944). The evolution of those ideas are explored by Rachman (1997) and by Prince (2018) who traced their influence specifically on interpersonal psychoanalysis.

Thompson's (1953) essay *Transference and Character Analysis* differentiates between transference and character resistance, incorporating both the concepts of Fromm and Sullivan. She describes a patient, who repeatedly becomes involved with married men who the patient claims are afraid to leave their wives. She says,

> This woman came to the conclusion that all men are cowed and browbeaten, but on each occasion, she had to try to be different from the wife by being helpful, making no demands, not making the usual fuss

about neglect. . . . This proved to be the childhood pattern of her relation to her father. A secret love existed between them but her mother
continued to dominate the father. The same was true of her lovers. She
was the preferred one, but none of them was free to affirm his love. . . .
Once we would have said . . . this woman relives her oedipus situation over and over again. But to call it a simple automatic reliving is
to overlook its dynamics. What function does it serve in her present
life . . . instead of a simple transference of a situation from the past, we
have a kind of character development, which is not resolved by simply recalling its origin. The patient has to work out all the subsequent
defensive maneuvers she developed in the course of growing in order
to protect herself from being hurt.

(Thompson, p. 266)

In this vignette, we hear the influences of both Fromm's notion of character
types and Sullivan's ideas about defensive operations in an original clinical
formulation by Thompson that is the hallmark of interpersonal psychoanalysis. She asks, "[W]hat function does it serve in her present life."

Interested in patterns of interaction within the whole field of reference,
Thompson was impressed by the work of Hanna Colm (1955), who spoke
of psychoanalysis in terms of field theory. Colm viewed, "the analytic
situation in terms of a mutual human relation" (p. 173). Those ideas are
clearly stated in Thompson's (1956), *The Role of the Analyst's Personality
in Therapy*, where she quotes Colm,

The analyst brings to the situation his whole past, that is, all of his
ways of relating, and his field gradually begins to interact with the
patient's field. At first, the analyst encounters the fringe areas of the
patient, i.e., his defenses, but eventually the center area of both is
reached. Her assumption is that the center area of the patient can be
reached only by a center reaction of the analyst. By his awareness
of his own spontaneous reactions, he becomes aware of the needs
and motives of the patient. The patient, on his part, experiences
acceptance and can, therefore, relate with his center (or core) reaction. The total personality of the analyst affects the total personality
of the patient.

(p. 173)

Thompson maintained her focus on the coming together of the total personality of the analyst and patient in their psychoanalytic work. It is what she taught, and it is what some of those who worked closely with her continued (see Levenson, 1989; Wolstein, 1994). Over time, she expanded and refined this approach in concert with her colleagues, yet she does not seize any credit for herself; but, she made certain that Colm receives credit for her field theory idea. Thompson is always fair and generous.

The cross-fertilization of concepts between Thompson, Horney, Fromm, and Sullivan was indispensable. It was as if the foursome added some yeast to their intellectual mix, creating a synergy of influences that resulted in an American brand of psychoanalysis (Hirsch, 2014; Stern, 2015). It would be fair to say that they each shaped, modified, and transformed each other's way of thinking. Their joint power was so great that consideration over who should be seen as the leader of the interpersonal tradition—Thompson, Sullivan, or Fromm—is sometimes settled by offering joint credit.

The views of Horney and Fromm were decidedly feminist. They challenged Freud's embrace of patriarchal society. Both Fromm and Horney wrote about "pregnancy envy" in men. Fromm at the invitation of Horney lectured in Chicago on matriarchal systems (see Funk, 2000) and Horney published her book *Neurotic Personality of Our Time*.

Horney, Fromm, and here I add Freida Fromm-Reichman, were strongly influenced by the work of J.J. Bachofen's *Mother Right* (originally published in 1861) on the significance of women as mothers. Thompson was not. Fromm's understanding of Bachofen's matriarchal social system,

> as part of culture and related to every aspect of life. . . . Women, particularly mothers, favored a social system of freedom, equality and peaceful relations among citizens.
>
> (Ortmeyer, 1998, p. 26)

This distinction is addressed in a discussion of Thompson's psychology of women where Thompson steps outside the views of her peers.

Fromm too stepped outside mainstream psychoanalytic thinking. He loosened his connection with his classical psychoanalytic training, as he integrated the Marxist concepts that appealed to him intellectually. For him, key concepts wedded in patriarchal premises were less appealing within a longer view of history that included matriarchal societies (Friedman, 2013, pp. 47–49).

Instead, Fromm focused on character orientations and their specific consequences (see *Man for Himself*, 1947).

During this same period, Thompson (1947) published her essay, "Changing Concepts of Homosexuality in Psychoanalysis." Fromm's paper (written sometime in the 1940s) titled "Changing Concepts of Homosexuality"
was initially thought to be authored by Fromm. The similarity of these
papers led Rainer Funk to withdraw the paper from Fromm's list of publications,[7] giving credit to Thompson for the essay.

Her ideas on homosexuality are conflicted. To her credit, she does not
lean toward pathologizing, but she does not embrace the notion of sexual
variations either. Twentieth century theorists were confined by cultural
attitudes despite their own proclivities. Speaking about Sullivan, Blechner
(2005) concludes,

> Sullivan's homosexuality was integral to his clinical and theoreti-
> cal innovations. Because there has been so much anxiety and mys-
> tification about his homosexuality, the importance of his sexuality to
> his theory has also been obscured. And that may also be one reason
> why sexuality has had a hazy and sometimes neglected position in
> interpersonal and relational theory in general.
>
> (p. 3)

Where these psychoanalytic pioneers were able to make progress was
on the role of the analyst's personality in psychoanalysis. Hirsch (2014)
attributes to Ferenczi and Rank the introduction of analytic subjectivity,
then to Sullivan, Fromm, and Thompson, in that order, the systematic elaboration of "what became the Interpersonal school or tradition" (p. 1). This
sequence is typical despite the demarcation of Thompson's place in line
as Ferenczi's direct descendent. Historians never seem to know exactly
where to place her. The answer should be first for a number of reasons,
including the fact that she brought back Ferenczi's ideas to America and
developed them further with Sullivan and Fromm. She modestly explains:

> Sullivan was a more influential factor in my psychiatric life than any
> other person. Certainly, he has influenced my life over a longer period.
> He influenced my first thinking, and because of his influencing my
> first thinking, this was carried over into my other relationships, so
> that when I went to Ferenczi, I was already very much oriented in

Sullivan's way, and—when Fromm and Horney came along—we also were very much in the same line as Sullivan. In fact, I would not have gone to Ferenczi, because who would have the nerve to go to Budapest all alone, if Sullivan hadn't insisted that this was the only analyst in Europe he had any confidence in. Therefore, if I was going to go to Europe and get analyzed, I had just better go there. So, I went.

(Thompson, 2017, p. 19)

Her reflections underscore Sullivan's influence on her personal and intellectual life. She elaborates:

When Ferenczi was in the United States in 1926, Sullivan met him and found his thinking the most congenial to his own way of thinking of any of the analysts. At the same time, it would be an exaggeration to say that they influenced each other to any extent. Their contact was too brief, and each continued to develop without further communication with each other.

(Thompson, 1978, p. 491)

She does not address how her influence could have had an effect on them. Uncharacteristically, she acknowledges that her move to Budapest to undergo treatment with Ferenczi was very brave. She then sets it aside as if it was not her own doing. She was a few generations away from having the tools to fully understand her gender difficulties. She continues,

When I got to Ferenczi, I realized for the first time that we were really controversial; that what we were thinking was anathema because, almost from the beginning, I found that Ferenczi thought very much the way we did and, in fact, he accused me of stealing his ideas one time and he could not believe that Sullivan had developed a way of thinking that was so close to his own, without any collaboration. I really think that he thought I was not telling him the truth for a long time about that. . . . I think that Sullivan's thinking had a great influence on Horney when she came to the United States, and also on Fromm-Reichmann.[8] There is no doubt about Fromm-Reichmann, who went and worked with him for many years. But Horney, also, I think, was very much influenced by him in those first years when she was here. Fromm, of course because of his background, was already pretty well oriented in a way to our thinking, and so when he came to the United States, he just naturally got connected up with us also. Another person who was greatly influenced by Sullivan was [William] Silverberg. He came to Baltimore in 1930 and worked at Sheppard Pratt and in that way became interested in Sullivan's work, and he had been in Berlin . . . and was . . . a little bit more orthodox than the rest of us. Now this group formed into an informal social group, "scientific social," I guess you might call it, and we called ourselves the "Zodiac." The zodiac met every Monday night in a speakeasy in the early days, and later in a more legitimate place when it could be done. . . . Anyway, the things we started talking about then became organized into Sullivan's thinking.

(pp. 19–20)

Where Karen Horney focused on how individuals in our culture escape anxiety by becoming hypersocial or hyperindustrious, Thompson argued that they seek both affection and power and that those two needs can clash. Her colleague, Erich Fromm argued that if humans turned away from the dangers and responsibilities inherent in freedom, they would ultimately turn toward authoritarianism. As for Harry Stack Sullivan, he was focused on how individual interactions with other people, especially significant others, determined their sense of security and a sense of self. Clara Thompson placed her emphasis on understanding what went on between people in ways that would facilitate or impede growth in their relationships. These different but similar positions were a mutually advantageous combination for each member of the quartet.

Influence, Inspiration, Guidance

Thompson, Horney, Sullivan, and Fromm were influenced, inspired, and guided by the work of two anthropologists, Franz Boas's (1932) *Anthropology and Modern Life* and his student Edward Sapir, who studied the way language and culture influence each other. Sapir was a professor of anthropology at the University of Chicago when he met Sullivan in 1926. Sapir introduced Sullivan to the Chicago School of Thought, which included the work of George Herbert Mead[9] and Charles Cooley,[10] "whose concepts of mind, self, and society are building blocks from which Sullivan developed his interpersonal theory of personality" (Burton, 1998, p. 849). They also became devoted friends and colleagues until Sapir's death in 1939.

Elizabeth Capelle (1993) writes that "in their search for a more satisfactory understanding of the psychological mechanisms of the 'tyranny of culture,' the culture-and-personality anthropologists had begun to investigate psychoanalysis" (p. 245). She notes that

> They found willing collaborators in Harry Stack Sullivan, Karen Horney, Erich Fromm and Clara Thompson, the analysts who were to become known as the "cultural school." The two groups had been brought together through the agencies of Sullivan, who since meeting Sapir in 1926 had been a fervent advocate of interdisciplinary collaboration.
>
> (pp. 247–248)

It is difficult to apportion ideas when they are in motion between people. Each idea can be an indirect guide to something new. Between Thompson, Sullivan, Fromm, and Horney there was a reciprocity, commitment, and creativity. They imported sociology and American cultural anthropology into psychoanalysis, aiming to sweep away notions of inherent human nature and inherent national, racial, or sexual characteristics (Wake, 2011). Fromm focused on the need for freedom and the need for belonging, Horney on the needs for affection and approval, and Sullivan on anxiety as a threat to loss of sense of security, while Thompson focused on the analytic encounter and the cultural pressures on women. As she describes this period:

> In the late 1920s, psychoanalysts began to concern themselves with character analysis, and a few years later, some analysts became interested in the study of comparative cultures and in the application of the findings of modern anthropology to the study of the development of human personality. Fromm and Sullivan became outstanding contributors in both of these fields, and each has his own unique contribution to the subjects.
>
> Thompson (1964a, p. 95)[11]

Thompson, Sullivan, Fromm, and Horney, Early Influences

Thompson was shaped by her American education, including the faculty at Pembroke/Brown University and Johns Hopkins School of Medicine. Fromm's strongest influence came from his time in Berlin studying sociology (Funk, 2000). Horney's biographer suggests that while she trained in Germany with Abraham and Sachs and was a founding member of the Berlin Psychoanalytic Institute, she was most influenced by her role as mother of three girls. Motherhood gave Horney an opportunity to observe the development of girls and their interests and concerns about their bodies. Unlike Freud, she made direct observations on the development of normal baby girls (Rubins, 1978). Sullivan drew enormously from the social scientists at the University of Chicago (Perry, 1982) in developing his ideas.

The psychoanalytic culturalists Thompson, Sullivan, Horney, and Fromm were influenced by Boas, Sapir, Benedict, and Mead, as they embraced a view of human behavior based on social behavioral patterns as well as biology. They shared a belief that the causes and treatment of mental problems could be understood as problems in living resulting from a conflict with cultural patterns. It is Thompson who served as the link between Ferenczi and Sullivan, though she would have felt it brash to promote herself as such.

Thompson, Horney, Fromm, and Sullivan each drew from their colleagues Margaret Mead and Ruth Benedict, who also influenced American psychoanalysis in their identification of culture as "the learned ways of behavior of a group" (Benedict, 1959, p. 12). Benedict said of the relationship of the individual to culture that, "The life history of an individual is first and foremost an accommodation to the patterns and standards traditionally handed down in his community" (pp. 2–3). Capelle noted that Mead (1935) used a similar "approach to the question of male and female nature in her book *Sex and Temperament*, the first systematic anthropological treatment of the subject" (1993, p. 262).

> Mead concluded from the diversity of behavior she observed in her study of several primitive cultures that there was no such thing as generic male or female nature, that instead "the personalities of the two sexes are socially produced."[12] The implication that Mead and

Benedict were careful to draw from these studies was that of the plasticity of human beings and their institutions; people could change, indeed, whole cultures could change.

(p. 263)

In recognition of those ideas, Thompson (1942) wrote:

The importance of cultural influences in personality problems has become more and more significant in psychoanalytic work. A given culture tends to produce certain types of character. . . . Most of these neurotic trends are found working similarly in both sexes.

(1942, p. 331)

Sullivan

Harry Stack Sullivan was the child of Irish Catholic immigrants. He grew up in an upstate New York farming community, where anti-Catholic, anti-Irish prejudice flourished. His mother resented his father, a hired hand, and felt she had married beneath her Irish family's status. He was a superior student although lonely and introspective. In high school, like Thompson, he was at the top of his class, its valedictorian. He moved on to Cornell to study physics, but his grades there were fair to poor. Eventually, he was dropped for failure to complete his work. Perry (1982) speculates that,

he probably lost his scholarship at Cornell because of his scholastic failure, and his consequent financial hardship might explain his inability to continue his education there or at any other undergraduate college.

(p. 25)

That he was a young gay man in Cornell's elitist sea of heteronormativity has not been sufficiently explored. One can envisage the difficulty he had fitting in and the isolation he experienced because of the homophobia he encountered both in himself and in others. Even his biographer Perry (1982) failed to fully acknowledge Sullivan's homosexuality despite being publicly documented by Chapman (1976), who declared "Sullivan was a homosexual, and this fact was well known to, or strongly suspected by, most of his contemporaries" (p. 12). Perry even felt she had to guard the names of Sullivan's friends for fear she would damage their names presumably if their homosexuality was revealed. For a fuller account of the harm done by Sullivan's biographers, see Vande Kemp (2004).

Despite his emotional suffering, Sullivan had the fortitude to enroll in the Chicago College of Medicine and Surgery and to find gainful employment to meet his tuition costs. The Chicago College of Medicine and Surgery had no clinic or hospital. Perry (1982) explains that his medical school training was average for that period. Sullivan never completed his college education; he did earn a professional degree in medicine, but he referred to the Chicago school he attended with contempt, calling it a "diploma mill" that granted medical degrees based on the payment of tuition rather than scholastic performance (Perry, 1982, p. 157). He received his license to practice medicine in 1918, two years before Thompson graduated from the leading medical school in the country. 1918 was also the year of the Spanish flu pandemic that resulted in school cancellations, boarded-up businesses, and in one month the death of nearly 200,000 people in the United States. These conditions were the backdrop of Sullivan's first two years of psychiatric training, which he spent first at St. Elizabeth's and then at Sheppard-Pratt. How each of them survived the pandemic and its aftermath is not discussed by biographers. Perhaps after the pandemic ebbed, so did the traumatic memories.

In Chicago, Sullivan was part of a broad social network of anthropologists, sociologists, and psychoanalysts, including Lionel Blitsten, a leading psychoanalyst in Chicago, and Dorothy Blitsten, whose book *Human Social Development* (1971) examined broadly the concerns of social bonds. Karen Horney lived around the corner from the Blitstens, and they became good friends. Lionel Blitsten and Dorothy Blitsten were important allies for Sullivan.

Thompson and Sullivan were both influenced by the teachings of Adolf Meyer, William Alanson White, and Edward Kempf. Perry (1982) suggests that by 1927 Sullivan was promoting the idea that he could improve the lives of his mostly young gay male patients' mental health by improving their "interpersonal relationships" (p. 7). At the same time, Thompson was sharpening her clinical skills in her private practice. By 1929, the Bulletin of the International Psychoanalytic Association lists Thompson and Sullivan as members of the American Psychoanalytic Association. Horney was then a member of the German Psychoanalytical Society, and in 1930 Erich Fromm was elected an associate member (Roazen, 2001).

Emotionally, both Sullivan and Thompson were detached, anxious, and lonely people. They were drawn to each other on multiple levels. It is unimaginable to think that they did not exchange letters during Thompson's absence in Budapest, but their letters have yet to be found.

Sullivan was given a free rein to treat "schizophrenics" in a ward at the Sheppard-Pratt, where he developed his ideas about clinical treatment. He was interested in the emotional problems of the young male schizophrenics and had modified the classical Freudian treatment method. He came to believe that his male patients were like him, in that they had missed an important developmental phase of chumship and acceptance. He designed the hospital environment around the belief that he could provide that missed experience (Blechner, 2005; Wake, 2011). With a similar inclination toward a missed developmental step, Ferenczi thought patients needed to be given the love they had missed as children (Rachman, 1997). Thompson (1944) wrote:

> Ferenczi believed that the child became ill as a result of the neurosis of his parents. "There are no bad children. There are only bad parents," he said. He firmly believed that a person became ill because of what had happened to him. In this, he claimed that he was reviving Freud's early idea of infantile sexual trauma. Actually, however, Ferenczi's concept was more broad than Freud's earlier one. Not only did he consider early sexual experiences as significant in producing traumata, but he viewed many attitudes of parents toward their children as traumatic. Expressing the feeling that children especially suffered as a result of the insincerity of parents, he said, "Children know the truth because they learn the meaning of words. After they learn the meaning of words, they become confused."
> (pp. 246–247)

Thompson goes on to explain Ferenczi's understanding of a problematic development:

> His idea was that, if a mother basically rejects her child, the child somehow knows it. After he learns words, he is told that mother loves him. What is he to believe? Ferenczi thought that because the child intuitively seems to know that the words are lies, he also may become a liar, assuming that that is the way to get along in life; or he may begin to doubt his own powers of observation. Ferenczi also believed that love is as essential to a child's healthy growth as food. With it

the child feels secure and has confidence in himself. Without it, he becomes neurotically ill.

(p. 247)

Thompson explains further:

[O]ther analysts, notably Fromm and Sullivan, have presented similar ideas, but I believe Ferenczi was quite alone in Europe around 1926 in this type of thinking. Unfortunately, these ideas were never published in any organized way. They crept into his ideas about technique; but, for the most part, they were simply notions that he communicated to his pupils.

(p. 247)

Silver (1993) notes how Ferenczi's impact on psychoanalytic work with the severely mentally ill has been too little acknowledged. She writes,

Expecting to find frequent references to Ferenczi in the transcripts of the nearly 100 lectures Sullivan gave at Chestnut Lodge, I was astounded to find that Sullivan at no time discussed, and only rarely alluded to, anyone who had contributed to his thinking. . . . Ferenczi is only occasionally mentioned in the various books on psychoanalytic treatment of the severely ill. With the discounting of his perspective went reading his papers, and yet very many of his ideas resurfaced, in the area of interpersonal therapy and in the British object relations school.

(p. 647)

Sullivan tirelessly promoted psychiatry, writing (letter Sullivan to Blitsten, 1940a) to his good friend Dorothy Blitsten:

I believe that we are going to get psychiatry on the map with considerable speed and measurable precision. Under the Selective Service System, all local examiners are being instructed to the effect that personality factors are significant, that they are not wholly mysterious, and that psychiatrists on the Advisory Board should be used freely. Sullivan worked toward the integration of the methods of psychiatry particularly his approach to understanding personality, into mainstream thinking in order to reduce world tensions and conflicts.

(Sullivan, 1940a)

In the same letter, Sullivan also counsels Dorothy Blitsten about her marriage sharing his thoughts on sexual intimacy in relationships:

A perfectionist might be willing to forego everything, if there was any imperfection. A person lost in psychoanalytic thinking might feel that the absence of lustful rapport indicated that everything was wrong. Both of these attitudes seem to me tedious in the extreme.

Sullivan was practical, empathic, and forthright in the way he counsels his friend.

Fromm

Like Thompson, Fromm grew up in a restrictive religious community. He later described his Orthodox Jewish community as having a "medieval atmosphere" (Funk, 2000, p. 8). For a time, like Thompson, he dreamed of a religious vocation, studying the Talmud and following in the footsteps of other men in his family. In his 20s, he came to reject Orthodox Judaism but always identified with the Judaic value of studies. He attended a notable German Jewish school and graduated with distinction. He became Zionist and by 1919 had founded an Association for Jewish People's Education in Frankfurt, which in turn established a Free Jewish Teaching Institute, where Martin Buber came to lecture. Fromm received a PhD in sociology from Heidelberg University and trained as a psychoanalyst under Frieda Reichmann, whom he married in 1926. He became friends with Georg Groddeck[13] from Baden-Baden, a close friend to both Ferenczi and Freud. Fromm admired Groddeck and was drawn to his ideas about psychosomatic medicine. Later as an avowed Marxist, he came to renounce Zionism and supported the struggle for the rights of the Palestinians. He joined the largely Marxist Frankfurt Institute for Social Research in 1930 and continued in the Institute when it migrated to the United States in 1933. He was influenced by Max Horkheimer, Hegel, Marx, and Max Weber. Fromm used the idea of 'social character' as a link between the individual unconscious and society.

Horney

Karen Horney too was raised in a rigid religious environment. Her father was stern, righteous, and religious (Rubins, 1978). His Evangelical creed ruled the home. As an avid reader, she escaped her family through books. She attended a *Klosterschule* (a type of convent school, though Protestant) in Hamburg, Germany that laid heavy emphasis on the history of religion, Bible study, theology, philosophy, literature, and languages. The sciences were avoided because of religious principles.

Like Thompson, Horney decided early that she wished to study medicine. The only school that could provide her with the necessary courses for medicine was the *Realgymnasium* for girls (Rubins, 1978). There she began to question her religious upbringing and was disappointed in her teachers. She went on to attend medical school at the University of Freiburg, the first German university to admit women. A young girl like Horney had few choices about where to live during her training so her mother decided to live with her while she went to school. In 1909, she married and moved to Berlin to complete her training. She struggled with the conflicting roles of professional woman, mother, and wife.

In order to practice medicine in Europe, a physician needed a medical doctorate degree after finishing medical school and passing the state medical examination. That meant locating a sponsor and accumulating case material or clinical training for a thesis. Horney received her clinical training at Berlin's Charité University Hospital in both the highly regarded neuropsychiatric services and the in-patient service of Professor Karl Bonhoeffer (Rubins, 1978). Horney was a few years older and ahead of Thompson professionally. The year after Thompson finished college Horney delivered a talk to the 22 members of the Berlin Psychoanalytical Society, entitled "Contribution to the Female Castration Complex" (Rubins, 1978).

Uniquely Thompson: The Analytic Relationship

On the topic of the analytic relationship, Thompson affirmed the mutually influential aspects of the analytic encounter. She differentiated herself from Ferenczi on the need for love as she distinguished a need from a demand for love (Thompson, 1943). This contribution to the analytic canon has not received appropriate acknowledgment; instead, it has been absorbed into contemporary practices. In an early paper, Thompson (1938b) traces the development of transference in a detached patient. The transference was altered when the patient realized the difference between his idea of the analyst and the new characteristics he encountered in the analyst. She utilizes a definition of transference as a reaction that comes from the patient's own past or life situation, expanded to include the fact that every patient possesses a mixture of "some ability to judge the analyst in reality mixed with much irrational evaluation" (p. 300). She would affirm that not everything is transference.

Thompson did not propose a need based, stage based self-system, or character styles in the same way as her other three colleagues Sullivan, Fromm, and Horney. Instead, her focus was on the therapeutic process itself. Each of these culturalists saw the role of anxiety in human behavior as central to development.

Her colleague Karen Horney (1937) argued that neurosis resulted from basic anxiety caused by interpersonal relationships. Horney's (1937) theory suggests that strategies used to cope with anxiety can be overused, causing them to take on the appearance of needs. Sullivan's (1940b) theory of anxiety took a similar path, arguing that personality is the result of strategies to decrease anxiety. Fromm (1941) argued that people's interactions with others, especially significant others, determine their sense of security, sense of self, and the dynamisms that motivate their behavior. In Thompson's (1950) review of theory and therapy, she traced the development of psychoanalysis from her perspective in her egalitarian manner, She ends her treatise saying,

> I have attempted to present the positive and negative aspects of the various theories and methods, keeping clearly in mind that psychoanalysis is still a science in its infancy and no school can lay claim to having discovered the final truth.
>
> (p. 243)

Thompson valued fairness and honesty as life's guiding principles.

Horney and Thompson were different from each other in the way they viewed the psychology of women. Thompson (2017)[14] said Horney, "seized upon . . . culturalist ideas to redirect the critique of Freud's theories of female sexuality that she had developed in the 1920s, her earlier work suggested that women were different from men, but nonetheless equal. Horney argued her points forcefully and publicly. By the end of the decade, she had published two books that extended her critique of Freud to his whole system, provoking a "landslide of anger" in the New York Psychoanalytic Society. (p. 19)

Thompson (2017) thought of herself as "a little less belligerent" than Horney (p. 9).

While Thompson agreed with many of Sullivan's ideas, she took sharp exception to his conception of the self-system in *Concepts of the Self in Interpersonal Psychoanalysis* (1958):

> Sullivan stated that the self-system tends to be relatively rigid and not easily modifiable by experience. In my opinion, he cannot have meant that the total self is relatively rigid. There seem to be all degrees of flexibility in it. Characteristics which have never encountered either strong approval or disapproval may change easily under the impact of new circumstances or even from further growth within. Characteristics, the disturbance of which produces only mild anxiety, may be fairly easily changed; but most people have a more or less extensive rigid portion, which has been developed in response to intense threat of anxiety. This, as I have said, includes defenses against impulses or activities found to be unacceptable to the significant people at some time during the course of development. Any attempt to modify this produces anxiety . . . is rigidly resisted . . .
>
> Sullivan seems usually to be thinking of this latter group of traits as the self-system . . . he pays no attention to other aspects of the self. . . . He talked a great deal about security operations. . . . As far as I can see, these security operations are the chief activity of this more limited self-system. . . . Perhaps his failure to emphasize that there are varying degrees of anxiety contributing to the choice of traits in the self is due to the fact that his conclusions were drawn . . . from the study of grave personality disorder, i.e., schizophrenia . . . all movements are concerned with "do I please" or "am I rejected?" . . . the self would then be one long security operation. The fear of rejection would constantly dominate the picture. I doubt whether this is universally true. There must be many whose early lives were sufficiently secure to permit the development of large areas of the self without concern for approval

or disapproval. . . . I do not believe the self, in interpersonal theory, is entirely the product of the attempt to avoid anxiety, but it is . . . a product of the society in which it develops.

(1958, pp. 12–13)

Fromm held many basic ideas in common with Sullivan but wrote more specifically about Western culture. Thompson (1964) reiterates Fromm's position:

According to Fromm's view . . . man is the least instinct-ridden of all the animals; he has fewer pre-formed ways of reacting at birth than any other creature; he literally has to be taught how to live. It follows that most of his drives are actually created by his society; therefore, society not only curbs some needs, but also creates new needs. He sees, for example, the lust for power and the craving for submission as drives created by the social order. In his gradual evolution from his animal past, man has created his society and has in turn been created by it. In other words, man has a dynamic relation to society, changing the course of history, while being changed by it.

(p. 96)

Fromm's democratic values appealed to Thompson's sense of equality. She wrote:

I especially refer to his discussion of rational and irrational authority, and of selfishness and self-love. He has pointed out that there are two types of authority. Genuine authority is based on competence. A person is an authority because he knows something the other does not know. In the course of imparting his knowledge to the other, his position of supe-riority diminishes as the listener or pupil also becomes competent. This, ideally, is the type of authority the analyst should have in his relation-ship to the analysand, and the parent to the child. In successful therapy, therefore, the analyst should in time lose his authoritative power, and the end goal should be one of equality between analyst and patient.

(1964, p. 98)

These thoughts may have resonated with Thompson's early immersion in the Free Baptist Church. Not for their religious convictions, they were not present in Fromm's thesis, but for the way he argued for fairness and equality. As noted earlier, Thompson and Fromm shared a set of moral principles that developed within their different religious communities, as did Horney and Sullivan.

In her comparison of Sullivan and Fromm, Thompson (1964d) maintained:

> Sullivan does not attempt to postulate what man might become in other circumstances. He observes him in this struggle. Because this is the field of his observation, he has only vague things to say about maturity (which he considers a rare phenomenon, at least in the experience of a psychiatrist). He has practically nothing to say about mature love. He does define what passes for love at the juvenile and preadolescent levels. Fromm, on the other hand, is much more concerned with the problem of maturity and with the ways in which man may succeed in transcending his culture. He defines maturity as the capacity for love and productive work, and he has much to say about them.
>
> Even with this point of difference, it seems to me that the thinking of the two men can supplement each other. That is, through Sullivan's approach, the person can learn of the forces which are molding him, often against his best interests, while Fromm's approach offers a constructive frame of orientation for future growth and a stimulus to transcend culture in search of what is good for man.
>
> In short, neither denies the importance of instinctual drives, but each believes they are relatively weak in the human and are not the usual cause of neurotic difficulty. Fromm's idea of the goal of therapy is somewhat more far-reaching than anything Sullivan has stated on the subject. According to Fromm, the goal of therapy is the transformation of the personality. This is achieved when the therapist succeeds in breaking through the defense systems and reaching the true core of the individual. In other words, one has exposed the true self. To roughly contrast the difference in therapeutic approach between Sullivan's methods and Fromm's, I would say that Sullivan concerns himself more with helping the patient to see how his defense machinery (security operations) works to the detriment of effective living, while Fromm attempts to cut through the defenses to communicate with the underlying constructive forces, leaving the security operations to fall by the wayside. The contributions of Sullivan and Fromm have come to be called the "cultural

school," because of the great emphasis of both on the interpersonal factors in personality formation and personal difficulties and the relative lack of emphasis on the more biologic drives as dynamic factors.

(pp. 199–200)

Thompson, Ferenczi, and Fromm on Love

Psychoanalytic views about love begin with Freud. But Freud's views on the topic, as Martin Bergmann (1988) explains, were focused on the past. He "ignored the place of hope in analysis and the phenomenon of loving" (p. 138). In the early days of psychoanalysis, analytic love was part of the language of libido, fused with innate drives connected to erogenous zones and transferred from one object to another. Whereas Ferenczi (1949) saw analytic love as primarily a non-erotic caring, a tender passion.

Clara Thompson describes her analysis in words that speak to an analytic love that fueled her emotional engagement. She compares her analysis with Ferenczi to,

> a happy childhood. . . . I didn't know what people were talking about around me—just like a child, it was, to live there in a country that was so foreign. I was really in a foreign country. I think of it as a time in which I came to—I was a very detached person before that, very schizoid, and I came to have relationships with people for the first time. In a comfortable social way. I still have difficulties with intimacy, although not too much.
>
> (Freud, 1952)

Bacciagaluppi (1989) suggests that Ferenczi's concept of love was the precursor to Fromm's therapeutic attitude. In his examination of Fromm's (1974) unpublished seminars, he points to Fromm's statement about the role of the analyst:

> The analyst understands the patient only inasmuch as he experiences in himself all that the patient experiences. Fromm writes of "productive relatedness between analyst and patient," of "being fully engaged with the patient, fully open and responsive to him," of "center-to-center

relatedness." Fromm concludes "the analyst must become the patient yet he must be himself."

(p. 231)

No study of analytic love is complete without reference to Thompson's friend and colleague Izette de Forest's *The Leaven of Love* (1954). de Forest both an analysand of Ferenczi's and Fromm's featured love as central to the psychotherapeutic process. She writes,

"Redemption by love" is a phrase used in appreciation by a perceptive patient to describe the psychotherapeutic genius of Sándor Ferenczi."

(p. 179)

She had hoped her book would provide a wider understanding of Ferenczi's insights. She argued there was a "similarity between the love given to a patient in psychotherapy with divine love, the evolving interpretation of which is traced throughout Biblical history" (p. xii).

de Forest was not a member of the inner circle of Fromm, Sullivan, Horney, and Thompson—the "social scientific" group as Thompson described it, but she was an important friend and colleague of Clara Thompson's. We learn from Brennan (2009) Thompson and de Forest met in San Moritz during the summer of 1929. There was "an exchange of ideas that proved fertile for them both" (p. 448). Reading over the correspondence between Thompson and de Forest, Brennan concludes that it, "[B]espeaks a closeness that seems to go beyond their simply being acquaintances" (p. 449). They were trusted friends.

Thompson agreed with de Forest on her evaluation of Ferenczi's work, taking exception to Ferenczi's idea of "making the analytic situation very dramatic" to increase its therapeutic value. Thompson (1943) argued:

I have serious doubts about the entire validity of the concept. I believe that the analytic situation, if not prevented from developing, will become dramatic and convincing by itself. Deliberately increasing the tension by withholding interpretation does not seem to me justified. I think interpretation can and should be so presented that it leads the patient to seek further. I would deal with resistance by discussing it rather than letting the patient act it out blindly and possibly to the point of despair. In not interpreting, the analyst is cooperating with the patient; e.g. in the case of the man to whom Mrs. de Forest said nothing for some time, it seems to me that she, by not explaining what he was doing, but simply reacting to it, had accepted his challenge and become involved in his feeling situation. In doing this, she certainly increased his anxiety, and I think in this anxiety unnecessary elements were added, such as doubt of the analyst on a reality basis. I think such a patient might well feel that his insecurity had been greatly increased.

(p. 65)

Her main disagreement with Ferenczi had to do with regression in the service of re-living an experience; a "therapeutic regression" to return emotionally to the experiences that originally produced the trauma (Rachman, 1997). Thompson did not accept the idea that actual trauma needed to be re-experienced to analyze it. Instead, she maintained:

It is my opinion that one of the most important functions of the analyst is to keep the patient in contact with reality. In the patient's most disturbed and irrational moments, he must be able to feel that the analyst is not deceived about reality. If, for example, he is attacking the analyst in rage, with strong feelings that the analyst has failed him or what not, he must be able to know with some remnant of rationality in himself that his accusations are not true, and that the analyst really wishes him well. The co-operative acting out on the part of the analyst, described by Ferenczi, can make the patient believe the analyst is really involved, and the function of reality testing is lost.

(1943, p. 66)

Thompson (1950) argued that what the patient needs is not love, but to "feel accepted and fundamentally respected" (p. 80). Her understanding sounds closer to Fromm's definition of a "productive relatedness between analyst and patient" (p. 75). She agreed with Fromm that "love does not manipulate the other person but shows respect and responsibility for him and the desire to see him grow and develop" (p. 75).

Thompson benefited from both of her analyses. She felt that her analysis with Ferenczi left her less troubled, more self-composed, and less withdrawn and that her analysis with Fromm "gave her more solidity."

In an interview in *Cosmopolitan* magazine, Thompson-Zolotow (1954) answers the question of why people seek analytic treatment. She draws attention to the conflicting values in society and to "an illness of the soul" as some of the reasons people seek treatment:

> It is clear that one cannot compromise with one's convictions for expediency's sake without suffering feelings of frustration and guilt. The psychotherapist's job is to help the patient understand the fears of isolation, loss of status, etc., which led him into the compromise, and to help him through insight, gain sufficient ego strength to live according to his convictions.
>
> (p. 194)

Similarly, Thompson (1959) speaks of "interpersonal difficulty" and isolation:

> The inability to make contact may be due to a hostile or even a destructive attitude. The individual feels so threatened by others that he must either drive them away or destroy them altogether . . . detached people who are not particularly hostile, who live as onlookers to life. They have an impersonal warmth so long as no closeness is involved, but they fear any entanglement of their emotions. They are lonely people, but unable to remedy their state through their own efforts.
>
> (p. 240)

While defending Ferenczi, she also elaborated on his shortcomings, not unlike the way Fromm talked about her faults:

> Certainly one might construe the idea of admitting one's fallibility to the patient as an invitation to a mutual analysis. To admit to a patient that one is wrong is one thing. To enter into extensive free association as to one's unconscious motives in making the error is quite another. Ferenczi at times was tempted to do the latter, and one could certainly interpret his ideas as endorsing the latter. This, in my experience, makes unwarranted demands on the patient and is not to his best interest. It is tantamount to turning to the patient for help and, although this

may flatter the patient, it puts a great burden of responsibility on him at the same time that it leaves him feeling unsupported himself. It may even lead him to feel he must suppress his own needs. However, the admission of a mistake can be evidence of strength. Then the aim of the statement is to correct a misconception and is made in the interest of clarifying the situation.

(Thompson, 1943, p. 65)

She insists further that:

Ferenczi's second point has also brought criticism and with some jus-tice. The difficulty lies in the definition of the word "love." I think Ferenczi was not entirely clear on this matter. His idea was that the analyst must give the patient all the love he needs. The basic need of every child is to be accepted, to feel himself secure with one indi-vidual. This type of acceptance is also what the patient needs. I think, however, Ferenczi tended to confuse the idea that the patient must be given all the love he needs with the idea he must be given all the love he demands. Obviously, the two are not identical. The neurotic individual after years of deprivation and frustration may develop an insatiable need of love. This is a complicated demand. Many emo-tions in no way connected with love are involved, such as exploiting others, getting revenge, power, etc. To satisfy this demand is not only humanly impossible, but, even if it would be satisfied, it is not thera-peutically valuable. However, I believe that the thing which Ferenczi was seeking, i.e. to give the patient the love he needs, is an important therapeutic discovery and that the mistakes he made in understanding the problem can be corrected.

(p. 65)

Thompson, Sullivan, Horney, and Fromm each situate anxiety as the force that leads to various defensive measures including avoidance, conformity, dissociation, and selective inattention, arguing these are moves to protect the self.

As a member of the cultural school of psychoanalysis, Thompson's ideas were fermented and grown in collaboration and discovery with her friends, Horney, Sullivan, and Fromm. With the help of her analysis with Erich Fromm, she hit her stride as a clinician, a leader, and a scholar.

Analytic Institutes became focused on the training of psychoanalysts and different schools of thought found homes within psychoanalytic societies and institutes. As Thompson rose to leadership roles in these societies and institutes, she played a formative role in the development of psychoanalysis in America. The next chapter opens with a view of Clara Thompson as a leader in her field including the organizational challenges she negotiated.

Notes

1 Letter Fromm to Crowley dated October 31, 1957, Erich Fromm Archive, Tubingen.
2 The 1979 paper was first written in 1956 and republished in *Interpersonal Psychoanalysis* in 1979.
3 It took until 1972, at a meeting of the American Psychiatric Association, for Dr. Anonymous to shake the foundations of the psychiatric community and announce that he was a psychiatrist and a homosexual.
4 See Rudnytsky, P. (2022), p. 139.
5 Clifford Read, dated Jan. 27, unpublished manuscript held at WAW archives.
6 Joseph D. Lichtenberg, MD, is Editor-in-Chief of *Psychoanalytic Inquiry*, Director Emeritus of the Institute of Contemporary Psychotherapy and Psychoanalysis, past President of the International Council for Psychoanalytic Self Psychology, and member of the Program Committee of the American Psychoanalytic Association. He has authored and edited numerous books and articles.
7 Personal communication Rainer Funk February 3, 2019. Dr. Funk is Director of the literary estate of Erich Fromm.
8 Frieda Fromm-Reichmann married Erich Fromm in and divorced him in. She moved into Chestnut Lodge and worked there for the rest of her career. She is the author of *I Never Promised You a Rose Garden*.
9 George Herbert Mead was an American sociologist and social theorist who argued the self is a product of social experience.
10 Charles Cooley, an American sociologist known for his concept that the self is an outgrowth of interpersonal interactions and perceptions of others.
11 The essay *Sullivan and Fromm* was written in 1956, published in Thompson's selected papers in 1964 and in Contemporary Psychoanalysis in 1979.
12 Mead (1935) wrote:

> The knowledge that the personalities of the two sexes are socially produced is congenial to every programme that looks forward towards a planned order of society. It is a two-edged sword that can be used to hew a more flexible, more varied society than the human race has ever built, or merely to cut a narrow path down which one sex or both sexes will be forced to march, regimented, looking neither to the right nor the left. It makes possible a Fascist programme of education in which women are forced back into a mould that modern Europe had fatuously believed to be broken forever.
>
> (p. 289)

13 Georg Groddeck was a German physician and director of the clinic at Baden-Baden.
14 Thompson presented "The History of the William Alanson White Institute," March 15, 1955, for the Harry Stack Sullivan Society. The talk was published in 2017 in *Contemporary Psychoanalysis*.

References

Bacciagaluppi, M. (1989). Erich Fromm's views on psychoanalytic "technique." *Contemporary Psychoanalysis, 25*(2), 226–243.

Bachofen, J. J. (1861) *Das Mutterrecht*. (Translator *D. Partenheimer*, 2008, *Mother Right*) Edwin Mellen Press, New York.

Bachofen, J. J. (1992). *Myth, religion and mother right*. Princeton: Princeton University Press.

Benedict, R. (1959). *Patterns of culture*. New York: Mariner Books.

Bergmann, M. (1988). On the fate of the intrapsychic image of the psychoanalyst after termination of the analysis. *Psychoanalytic Study of the Child, 43*, 137–153.

Blechner, M. J. (2005). The gay Harry Stack Sullivan: Interactions between his life, clinical work, and theory. *Contemporary Psychoanalysis, 41*(1), 1–19.

Blitsten, D. (1971). *Human Social Development*. College & University Press.

Boas, F. (1932). *Anthropology and modern life*. New York: W. W. Norton.

Brennan, W. (2009). Ferenczi's forgotten messenger: The life and work of Izette de Forest. *American Imago, 66*(4), 427–455.

Burton, K. (1998). Lucile Dooley, M.D. *Psychoanalytic Review, 85* (1), 51–73.

Capelle, E. L. (1993). Analyzing the "modern woman": Psychoanalytic debates about feminism, 1920–1950 (Unpublished doctoral dissertation). Columbia University.

Capelle, E. L. (1998). Clara Thompson as culturalist. *Psychoanalytic Review, 85*(1), 75–93.

Chapman, A. H. (1976). *Harry Stack Sullivan: His life and his work*. New York: Putnam Adult.

Colm, H. (1955). A field-theory approach to transference and its particular application to children. *Psychiatry, 18*(4), 339–352.

de Forest, I. (1954). *The leaven of love: A development of the psychoanalytic theory and technique of Sándor Ferenczi*. New York: Harper & Row.

Drescher, J. (2017). Smoke gets in your eyes: Discussion of "When Harry Met Jimmie." *Psychoanalytic Perspectives, 14*(1), 31–39.

Ferenczi, S. (1949). Confusion of the tongues between the adults and the child (The language of tenderness and of passion) (M. Balint, Trans.). *International Journal of Psychoanalysis, 30*, 225–230.

Freud, S. (1952). Interview with Clara Thompson (K. R. Eissler, Interviewer). Manuscript/mixed material. Sigmund Freud Papers: Interviews and

Recollections, Set A, 1914–1998 (Box 122). Manuscripts Division, Library of Congress, Washington, DC. www.loc.gov/item/mss3999001575

Friedman, L (2013). *The lives of Erich Fromm: Love's prophet* (Asst. Anke M. Schreiber). New York: Columbia University Press.

Fromm, E. (1933). *Neurotic personality of our time*. Norton Press, NY.

Fromm, E. (1941). *Escape from freedom* (US), *The fear of freedom* (UK). New York: Farrar & Rinehart.

Fromm, E. (1947). *Man for himself, an inquiry into the psychology of ethics.* Henry Holt & Co., New York.

Fromm, E. (1968, April 5). Letter to Ralph Crawley. The Oskar Diethelm Library, DeWitt Wallace Institute for the History of Psychiatry. The Weill Cornell Medical College, The Ralph Crowley Papers, Box 5, Fol. 7., New York, NY.

Fromm, E. (1974). *Transcript of ten unpublished seminars held in Locarno, Switzerland July 1974.* Tübingen: Erich Fromm Archives.

Funk, R. (2000). *Erich Fromm: His life and ideas*. New York: A&C Black.

Funk, R. (2019). *Life itself is an art: The life and work of Erich Fromm* (S. Kassouf, Trans.). New York: Bloomsbury Academic.

Hirsch, I. (2014). *The interpersonal tradition: The origins of psychoanalytic subjectivity.* London: Routledge.

Horney, K. (1937). *The neurotic personality of our time*. New York: W. W. Norton & Co.

Levenson, E. A. (1989). Whatever happened to the cat? Interpersonal perspectives on the self. *Contemporary Psychoanalysis, 25*(4), 537–553.

Mead, M. (1935). *Sex and temperament*. New York: Morrow.

Meigs, K. (2017). The failure of Clara Thompson's Ferenczian (Proxy) analysis of Harry Stack Sullivan. *The American Journal of Psychoanalysis, 77*, 313–331.

Moulton, R. (1975). Early papers on women: Horney to Thompson. *American Journal of Psychoanalysis, 35*(3), 207–223.

Ortmeyer, D. H. (1998). Revisiting Erich Fromm. *International Forum of Psychoanalysis, 7*, 25–33.

Oteri, D. (2013, May 16). Inside the Zodiac club: NYC's 145-year-old secret dinner society. *Gothamist*. Retrieved from https://gothamist.com/food/inside-the-zodiac-club-nycs-145-year-old-secret-dinner-society

Perry, H. S. (1982). *Psychiatrist of America: The life of Harry Stack Sullivan*, Belknap Press, Cambridge, MA.

Prince, R. (2018). The influence of Ferenczi on interpersonal psychoanalysis. In A. Dimitrijevic, G. Cassullo, & J. Frankel (Eds.), *Ferenczi's influence on contemporary psychoanalytic traditions*. pp. 206–212 London and New York: Routledge Press.

Rachman, A. W. (1997). *Sándor Ferenczi: The psychotherapist of tenderness and passion.* New York: Jason Arson.

Read, C. (Unpublished manuscript, January 27). Harry Stack Sullivan: A remembrance. William Alanson White Archive.

Roazen, P. (2001). The exclusion of Erich Fromm from the IPA. In *Publication of the International Erich Fromm Society* Gesellschaft. Alle Rechte vorbehalten.

Rubins, J. L. (1978). *Karen Horney: Gentle rebel of psychoanalysis*. New York: Dial Press.

Shapiro, S. (1993). Clara Thompson: Ferenczi's messenger with half a message. In *The legacy of Sándor Ferenczi*. Hillsdale, NJ: Analytic Press.

Silver, A. L. S. (1993). Countertransference, Ferenczi, and Washington, DC. *Journal of the American Academy of Psychoanalysis, 21*(4), 637–654.

Silver, A. L. S. (1996). Women who lead. *American Journal of Psychoanalysis, 56*(1), 3–16.

Stern, D. B. (2015). The interpersonal field: Its place in American psychoanalysis. *Psychoanalytic Dialogues, 25*(3), 388–404.

Sullivan, H. S. (1940a, November 27). Letter to Dorothy Blitsten. The Oskar Diethelm Library, DeWitt Wallace Institute for the history of psychiatry. The Weill Cornell Medical College, The Dorothy R. Blitsten Correspondence, Box 1, Fol. 1., New York, NY.

Sullivan, H. S. (1940b). *Conceptions of modern psychiatry*. The first William Alanson While Memorial Lectures. William Alanson White Psychiatric Foundation. New York: W. W. Norton & Company.

Sullivan, H. S. (1956). *Clinical studies in psychiatry*. William Alanson White Psychiatric Foundation. New York: Norton Library.

Thompson, C. (1938a). Notes on the psychoanalytic significance of the choice of analyst. *Psychiatry, I*, 295–216.

Thompson, C. (1938b). Development of awareness of transference in a markedly detached personality. *International Journal of Psychoanalysis, 19*, 299–309.

Thompson, C. (1942). Cultural pressures in the psychology of women. *Psychiatry, 5*(3), 331–339.

Thompson, C. (1943). "The therapeutic technique of Sándor Ferenczi": A comment. *International Journal of Psychoanalysis, 24*, 64–66.

Thompson, C. (1944). Ferenczi's contribution to psychoanalysis. *Psychiatry, 7*(3), 245–252.

Thompson, C. (1947). Changing concepts of homosexuality in psychoanalysis. *Psychiatry, X*, 183–189.

Thompson, C. (1950). *Psychoanalysis: Evolution and development*. New York: Hermitage House.

Thompson, C. (1953). Transference and character analysis. *Samiksa, 7*(4), 260–270.

Thompson, C. (1954, March). What you should know about psychiatry by Maurice Zolotow. *Cosmopolitan Magazine*.

Thompson, C. (1956). The role of the analyst's personality in therapy. *American Journal of Psychotherapy, 10*, 347–359.

Thompson, C. (1956–1957). *Letters to Erich Fromm*. Courtesy of Dr. Rainer Funk, Literary Estate of Erich Fomm, Erich Fromm Institute Tubingen.

Thompson, C. (1958). Concepts of the self in interpersonal theory. *American Journal of Psychotherapy, 12*(1), 5–17.

Thompson, C. (1959). The interpersonal approach to the clinical problems of masochism. In J. Masserman (Ed.), *Individual and familial dynamics* (pp. 31–37). New York: Grune and Stratton.

Thompson, C. (1964a). Sullivan and Fromm. In M. R. Green (Ed.), *Interpersonal psychoanalysis: The selected papers of Clara M. Thompson* (pp. 95–100). New York: Basic Books.

Thompson, C. (1978). Sullivan and psychoanalysis. *Contemporary Psychoanalysis, 14*(1), 488–501.

Thompson, C. (1979). Sullivan and Fromm. *Contemporary Psychoanalysis, 15,* 195–200.

Thompson, C. (2017). The history of the William Alanson White Institute. *Contemporary Psychoanalysis, 53*(1), 7–28.

Vande Kemp, H. (2004). Harry Stack Sullivan (1892–1949): Hero, Ghost, and Muse, in Stern, M. & Marchesani, R. (Eds). *Saints and Rogues: Conflicts and Convergence in Psychotherapy.* Routledge Press, New York.

Wheatland, T. (2009). *The Frankfurt school in exile.* Minnesota: University of Minnesota Press.

Wolstein, B. (1994). The evolving newness of interpersonal psychoanalysis: From the vantage point of immediate experience. *Contemporary Psychoanalysis, 30*(3), 473–499.

Chapter 2

Psychoanalytic Institutes and Societies

From Washington-Baltimore to
New York City

Key US East Coast Organizations and Key Figures

1909   Freud visits America at Clark University, MA.
1911   The New York Psychoanalytic Society (NYPS) established, founded by Abraham A. Brill.
1911   The American Psychoanalytic Association (APsaA) established by Ernest Jones, Adolf Meyer, and others.
1922   NYPS held its first series of lectures.
1923   NYPS Educational Committee formally organized the Society's teaching functions.
1926   Informal society formed in Washington-Baltimore, Thompson, and others.
1930   Washington-Baltimore Psychoanalytic Society formed; Thompson elected president. (Accredited by APA in 1932, affiliated with International Psychoanalytical Association[1])
1931   New York Psychoanalytic Institute established, Sandor Rado, Educational Director.
1933   William Alanson White Foundation, Harry Stack Sullivan, Founder.
1936   Washington School of Psychiatry, Harry Stack Sullivan, Founder.
1939   New York Psychoanalytic Institute, walk out in support of Karen Horney.
1940   Washington-Baltimore Psychoanalytic Institute; Lewis Hill Director (The Training program of Washington-Baltimore Psychoanalytic Society).

DOI: 10.4324/9781003284840-3

1941   The Association for the Advancement of Psychoanalysis, William Silverberg president, Clara Thompson, Vice-President, Harold Kelman, Secretary and Stephen Jewett, treasurer.

1941   American Institute for Psychoanalysis, Karen Horney, Dean.

1943   New York arm of Washington School of Psychiatry (to become the William Alanson White Institute), Harry Stack Sullivan, Clara Thompson, Erich Fromm, Frieda Fromm-Reichmann.

1944   New York Medical College, Stephen Jewett, Department Chair.

1946   William Alanson White Institute, Clara Thompson, Director, Erich Fromm Clinic Director. (Baltimore Psychoanalytic Society, Waelder-Hall; Washington Psychoanalytic Society, Sullivan).

1951   William Alanson White Institute of Psychiatry, Psychoanalysis, and Psychology, Clara Thompson, Director.

1956   American Academy of Psychoanalysis, The first president of the Academy was Janet Rioch Bard.

This chapter tells the story of Thompson's involvement in psychoanalytic training institutes and societies. In America, the path to becoming a psychoanalyst followed the Eitingon or European Model consisting of three elements defined within an analytic training institute, a personal analysis, a didactic curriculum, and supervised clinical work (Hale, 1995). As Thompson concluded in 1958, training institutes and their associated graduate societies can generate a sense of home though, for many, they can become the site of rivalries, hostilities, and conciliatory tactics where struggles to define and elaborate what constitutes "psychoanalysis" and importantly who can practice it take place:

> I believe that one inner cause for the tendency of an institute to become a home is the objective power which the training analyst has in the real life situation of his trainee, which facilitates the acting-out of the transference situation rather than resolving it. This leads to a flourishing of rivalries and hostilities or appeasing and ingratiating tactics on the part of the trainee.
>
> (Thompson, 1958, p. 49)

Thompson (2017) explains her place in this psychoanalytic history:

> The Berlin Institute and the Vienna Institute were the two first institutes of psychoanalysis [1918]. Later there came London and Budapest. I think that I have the distinction of being the only American medical person who was analyzed in Budapest. There were many analysts in the United States who were analyzed by Ferenczi, but they were all Hungarians who have come here since their analysis. I think I am the only medical person from the United States who went over there to be analyzed. Therefore, I did not have the experience that the people who went to Berlin and Vienna had having courses, because all the courses in Budapest were given in Hungarian, and I was not very proficient at that. There were, however, several non-medical people from the United States who were analyzed by Ferenczi and have become analysts. I suppose the best known one to us here is Izette de Forest, who was analyzed just a little before I was. I think she suffered from both kinds of treatment of Ferenczi, both the deprivation and the relaxation therapy. But I escaped the deprivation.
>
> (pp. 14–15)

While Clara Thompson was not present at the dawn of the discipline in America, she was involved in the field early in its development. A quick look back shows that discussions of the discipline surfaced the same year as Thompson's birth and the year *Studies in Hysteria* was first issued.[2]

In 1893, a New England physician, Robert. T. Edes, gave a lecture to the Massachusetts Medical Society and mentioned Breuer and Freud's ideas on suppression (Burnham, 1956, p. 66). William James too is said to have mentioned the Breuer–Freud studies as early as 1894 in his lectures at Harvard. And, in 1896 an abstract of Freud's paper on the etiology of hysteria was published in the *Journal of the American Medical Association* (Burnham, 1956). This early interest in psychoanalysis pre-dates the often-cited arrival of psychoanalysis to America in 1909, when Freud accepted G. Stanley Hall's invitation to lecture at Clark University (Evans & Koelsch, 1985),[3] accompanied by Ferenczi and Jung and attended by 175 educators, physicians, and other notable people.

Clara Thompson was 18 in 1911, the year both The New York Psychoanalytic Society (NYPS) was founded by Abraham A. Brill and The American Psychoanalytic Association (APsaA) was founded by her soon-to-be mentor, Adolf Meyer with the support of Ernest Jones and Sigmund Freud.[4] According to Hale (1995) in 1917, "[T]wo small professional psychoanalytic organizations" existed in America led by neurologists and psychiatrists; one was "an eclectic "American" version and the other a "more orthodox Freudian practice" (Hale, p. 6).

The orthodox Freudian group, NYPS, held its first series of lectures in 1922 and in 1923 and created an educational committee to formally organize the Society's teaching functions. The educational model of NYPS was based on the European tripartite model. Two of the major controversies within psychoanalytic organizations centered on whether to permit the training of non-medical individuals, or lay analysts as they were called, and how to reconcile the different approaches to psychoanalytic training (Benveniste, 2006).

Thompson graduated from Johns Hopkins Medical School in 1920. There were clinical requirements for the degree that included an internship and residence. At Johns Hopkins, she worked as a house officer and a psychiatric intern and she did a rotating internship at the New York Infirmary for Women and Children before returning to Baltimore for a three-year residency in psychiatry at the Phipps Clinic under Adolf Meyer. American psychiatry then was a mix of Adolf Meyer's psychobiology with various psychoanalytic models.[5]

It was during her second year of residency in 1923 that she met Harry Stack Sullivan. In her third year, Adolf Meyer put her in charge of his private patients while he was away. That year, at the age of 31, she also underwent her first psychoanalytic treatment with Joseph Cheesman (Snake) Thompson. As Green (1964) describes it,

> Her classmates, who had always known her as rather bitterly unhappy and alone, were impressed with the great rapport that she had with her analyst. The two of them were frequently seen dining together or, walking arm in arm, talking animatedly. For Clara, this must have been a precious relief from the burdens of her loneliness and unhappiness.
>
> (p. 353)

By 1925, Clara Thompson and Adolf Meyer locked horns over her choice of her psychoanalyst Joseph Thompson who Meyer detested. Meyer pressured Clara Thompson to stop seeing him. She refused and in the middle of controversy resigned her position (see *Clara M. Thompson's Early Years and Professional Awakening: An American Psychoanalyst (1893–1933)*.)

By that time, Clara Thompson had started a private practice in Baltimore and did some teaching to supplement her income. Green (1964) reports that a classmate who remains nameless had not seen her for several years remarked:

> I found a new and unsettling world surrounding her. Freud encircled us, on the bookshelves, in conversation, in our social life—all her friends were psychiatrists or psychoanalysts. . . . I spent a few hours in analysis with her, merely scratching the surface, but giving me some insights which changed the whole course of my life.
>
> (p. 354)

Clara Thompson had moved into a leadership position in 1930 as President of the Washington-Baltimore Psychoanalytic Society. There she participated in the teaching and training of psychoanalysts. From the outset, she was involved with other luminaries in psychiatry, psychoanalysis, anthropology, and sociology, all interested in clinical psychoanalysis and human development. The history of organizational psychoanalysis is riddled with competition, controversy, demands for loyalty, and betrayal. Frosch (1991) describes how he borrowed the title for his essay *The New York Psychoanalytic Civil War* from "Jones's (1934) characterization of "the schisms in America as the *American Psychoanalytic Civil War*" (p. 1037). Frosh offers a valuable description of the events.

However, Thompson gave her own account of this history in 1955 at the Harry Stack Sullivan Society (Published in 2017). As she explains it, beginning in 1926 she was involved with an informal society that began to meet regularly in the Washington-Baltimore area (Noble & Burnham, 1969). The group's membership included clinicians who were interested in psychoanalysis including Lewis Hill, Eleanora Saunders, Majorie Jarvic, Bernard Robbins, and William Silverberg. She recalls, "The group disbanded, and a new society was formed in 1930, known as the Washington-Baltimore Psychoanalytic Society" (p. 15). While the group was founded by Harry Stack Sullivan, they elected Clara Thompson to serve as its first president. This was the start of a non-Freudian, non-classical psychoanalysis that later was branded as interpersonal psychoanalysis.

Then in 1936, Harry Stack Sullivan founded the Washington School of Psychiatry, with a focus on teaching and research and training in psychodynamic theory, psychoanalysis, the social and biological sciences, and the study of the contribution of culture in human development. This "eclectic" relatively small group of people established a non-Freudian psychoanalytic training tradition that included new theories and clinical practices. This history is an amazing story with many twists and turns that are only briefly touched on here.

Meanwhile, the more orthodox analysts had established the New York Psychoanalytic Institute in 1931 and patterned itself after the Berlin Psychoanalytic Institute. Sandor Rado[6] was its first educational director.[7]

"An Institute Is Not a Home"

Thompson learned many lessons over the course of her career not the least of which is that an institute is not a home. In November of 1957, she delivered a warning about training institutes: Excessive orthodoxy and power dynamics in institutes can cause different kinds of intimidation, and idealization. Watch out she warned for rivalries and hostilities, appeasing and ingratiating tactics, greed, and opportunism. In her paper entitled "An Institute Is Not a Home: A Study of the Emotional Climate of Psychoanalytic Institutes" she begins by reassuring her audience that although the title may make it sound "frivolous," the subject matter is quite a "serious" problem in analytic institutes. She jokes, maybe, a better title would have been, "An Institute Is in Danger of Becoming Too Much of a Home."

Edgar Levenson (personal communication 2021) recalled that the title alludes to a book by a famous madame, Polly Adler, *A House Is Not a Home*. Adler ran a brothel at The Majestic Hotel, 215 West 75th Street.[8] Thompson's use of this title shows her charming side and sense of humor. One can imagine the audience giggling when she announced the paper's title.

In 1958, she published that same paper as "*A Study of the Emotional Climate of Psychoanalytic Institutes*." Thompson with her now-serious title turns attention to the organizational structure of psychoanalytic institutes where the education and training of the psychoanalyst take place. She views the power of the transferential relationships that develop within those communities as problematic. She provides her opinions about the power dynamics of excessive orthodoxy, intimidation, and idealization that precipitate as she sees it, a crisis in analytic training.

> I believe that one inner cause for the tendency of an institute to become a home is the objective power which the training analyst has in the real life situation of his trainee, which facilitates the acting-out of the transference situation rather than resolving it. This leads to the flourishing of rivalries and hostilities, or appearing and ingratiating tactics on the part of the trainee. I believe that these reactions are not quite so powerful when the training analyst has no voice in training decisions about his (sic) analysand. However, they are still in the same community and the tendency to act out rather than resolve the transference still takes place.
>
> (1958, p. 49)

She maintains that the close family group of an institute can become a toxic situation during training. She explains further,

> Wars and persecution tend to consolidate groups. When faced with a common enemy, bickering and small differences tend to fade away, or at least remain in abeyance for the time being. The early history of psychoanalysis was one of persecution. . . . The dissemination of psychoanalytic knowledge became a crusade.
>
> (p. 45)

The controversy of whether psychoanalysis is a crusade, a movement, or a cause settled on it being a profession (Eisold, 2003).

Thompson's experiences inside psychoanalytic training institutes led to her issuing cautions:

> [I]n . . . the psychoanalytic institute all the satisfactions and evils of a close family group seem to be revived again. The very way in which various groups are referred to indicates this trend . . . the Horney group . . . the Freudian group, and so on.
>
> (p. 45)

Her particular psychoanalytic family group began in the Washington-Baltimore area in the 1920s and 1930s with an evolving and complex mix of people, therapeutic ideas, and financial plans. It included pioneers in psychiatry: Adolf Meyer, William Alanson White, Harry Stack Sullivan,

Erich Fromm, Frieda Fromm-Reichmann, Karen Horney, and many other important players including Lucille Dooley, Edward Sapir, Harold Lasswell, Ernest Hadley, and William Silverberg, to name only a few. Many biographers and psychoanalytic historians have described this period (e.g., Chapman, 1976; Eisold, 2018; Frosch, 1991; Funk, 2000; Paris, 1994; Perry, 1982; Rubins, 1978).

By the time Thompson wrote *A Study of the Emotional Climate of Psychoanalytic Institutes* (1958), she had weathered many battles and placed a value on creating a space for independent psychoanalytic thinking for non-Freudian analysts. She knew full well that institutes and their societies often foster, in her words, "rivalries and hostilities, leading training candidates into appeasing and ingratiating tactics" (p. 49). Perhaps she hoped by issuing a warning—an institute was not a home—she might prevent a recapitulation of familial patterns in future generations of psychoanalysts within their institutes. She thought herself lucky that she had trained abroad and thus avoided those pitfalls thereby achieving independence:

> In some ways, we who were analyzed in Europe in the 1920s were fortunate. We had to leave our analysts and go to a far country. Some of my analysands have been similarly fortunate since in the last thirty years I have been a training analyst in four different institutes. They have been able to disagree with me on many theoretical points as well as becoming physically disentangled from my immediate environment.
>
> (pp. 50–51)

It is important to keep in mind what Thompson's cohort of psychoanalytic non-Freudian pioneers were trying to accomplish when they set themselves to establish training institutes. They were interested not only in the development of non-Freudian training but also in a model of therapy where the social context and culture are considered; a therapeutic model where the therapist does not stand at a distance from the patient in a cool detached manner but where an empathic connection and authenticity are valued; and where training institutes could teach analysts how to conduct and further their psychoanalytic knowledge without continually having to defer to Freud and his theories. Marylou Lionells, a past director of William Alanson White, believed that Thompson valued "the cooperation among institutions and the importance of avoiding parochialism," (Lionells, 2017, p. 38) yet she was also aware, as was Fromm, of how, "the crusading character of psychoanalytic groups is well expressed by what they call themselves—that is, the psychoanalytic *movement*. Other specialties are not spoken of as 'movements.' The word has a religious aura" (Thompson, 1958, p. 45).

Given her break from the religiousness of her family, the Free Will Baptists, she was averse to anything with a religious aura.

The Long Look: Telling and Retelling

Clara Thompson was one of the founders, along with Erich Fromm, Frieda Fromm-Reichmann, Harry Stack Sullivan, David Rioch, and Janet M. Rioch, and became the Director of the William Alanson White Institute in 1946. How the institute itself came into being is embedded in a complex history beginning with what we might think of today as a start-up. A new enterprise, The William Alanson White Psychiatric Foundation spawned innovative associations, schools, and institutes involving various participants.

As noted, Clara Thompson's first leadership position was in 1930 when she was elected President of the Washington-Baltimore Psychoanalytic Society. At the time, she was living in Baltimore and spending—the summers of 1928 (for two months), 1929 (for two months), 1930 (three months), before moving to Budapest for two years from 1931 to 1933.

A closer look into the period uncovers as many versions of the events as storytellers. One of the more colorful is a talk delivered on October 24, 1969, simply titled "Talk," by Dr. Dexter Bullard, Director of Chestnut Lodge, at the Sheppard and Enoch Pratt Hospital. Chestnut Lodge was originally founded by Bullards's father. Dexter Bullard graduated from Yale College, the year Clara Thompson completed medical school and then attained his medical degree from University of Pennsylvania. He trained in psychiatry at the Washington Psychoanalytic Institute and the Washington School of Psychiatry. His "Talk," a remembrance of Harry Stack Sullivan, delivers a historical perspective on psychoanalysis in America. My copy of the "Talk" is typed with handwritten corrections and dates inserted along the left margin. At the top is written, "Confidential not for distribution without Dr. Bullard's expressed permission." The transcription of "Talk" includes some questions by an unknown interviewer to whom Bullard responds. Along with his recollections of Harry Stack Sullivan, it covers the history leading up to the establishment of the White Institute.

Bullard, born in 1898, was five years younger than Thompson. He was an analysand of Sullivan. His (1969) recollections cover American psychoanalysis from the 1920s to 1940s. He describes the history of how the William Alanson White Institute came to be. He begins at the Maryland Psychiatric Society and the Washington-Baltimore Society when they were one entity. Bullard warns his audience that his recollections are out of order, but in the left-hand margin of the paper, the dates in sequence are noted, perhaps after the fact. According to the margin notations, Bullard begins in the 1920s:

> This is going to be quite out of any chronological order because I jotted down a few reminiscences about Harry yesterday afternoon while I actually had about fifteen minutes of unscheduled time. I don't remember when I first met Harry Stack. It was at St. Elizabeth's, But I don't recall the occasion of the meeting. The one very vivid memory of him was when Gregory Zilboorg came down to Phipps and read a paper on depression, and Adolf Meyer was to have been the principle discussant. I guess this was the Maryland Psychiatric Society—it was a good-sized group anyhow. It was here in Baltimore.

Bullard continues noting the key players—Sullivan, Hadley, White, Edward Sapir, Harold Lasswell, and Lucille Dooley—and maintains they "concocted" the William Allanson (sic) White Psychiatric Foundation in the School. Bullard adds

> Harry really had some grandiose notions. The money was to come from soliciting the families of prominent people that William A. White had seen and also that Sullivan had seen in the New York practice. . . . Harry cooked up a budget of $17,000.000. This was to be the endowment of the school. He was going to get $30,000. a year. Hadley was to get that much—I don't know how much Sapir and Lasswell we're going to get, but anyhow this was to be a built-in paid-up faculty so no one would have any financial worries . . . unhappily William A. White died before passing on the names of the people who were going to be tapped for this endowment fund.

One of Bullard's memories, concerns Clara Thompson, he writes:

> Once I was very curious as to who his [Harry Stack Sullivan] analyst had been and went at it in what I thought to be a very diplomatic way

and it turned out it wasn't. I said, "now you're doing a lot of supervision and you're doing a lot of training analyses and you know that the American requires that the training analyst to be accredited and have had his own personal analysis." Harry looked up and said "well if that question ever comes up, I will have no trouble in convincing the American Psychoanalytic Association of my credentials." End of investigative curiosity on my part. I am quite sure that at Sullivan's memorial service Clara Thompson did mention that. . . . I was there but I must have blocked it out because that was it was a most unusual service. They had a string quartet playing.

Bullard's recollections about the financial arrangements paint a picture of how the organizers of the William Alanson White Foundation imagined their new enterprise. There would be money to cover the salaries of key participants. The money would come from soliciting the patients and their families of both William Alanson White and Harry Stack Sullivan, a move that today would be considered unethical. Perry (1982) confirms the latter part of the financial history, adding that Sullivan and Hadley kept "these embryonic organizations going between 1939 and 1945, both financially and psychologically" (p. 357).

The William Alanson White Psychiatric Foundation

Despite the collapse of the original financing plans, by December 1933, the William Alanson White Foundation had a certificate of incorporation in hand. Sullivan became the first president of the Foundation. He, along with Lucile Dooley and Ernest E. Hadley, signed a certificate of incorporation. Perry (1982) explains:

> All three of them were active in the Washington-Baltimore Psychoanalytic Institute: Dooley was the president elect for 1934; Hadley was chairman of the training committee; and Sullivan was a member of the education committee. The Institute, a spin-off of the foundation, was not incorporated. The Foundation held the purse strings of the institute with Sullivan as a critical link between the two groups.
>
> (p. 360)

The Foundation was the sponsor for the Washington School of Psychiatry and the journal *Psychiatry*.

A Foundation With Double Vision

Sullivan's vision for the Foundation was different from his colleagues, Hadley and Dooley. Sullivan saw psychiatry as essential but sociology, anthropology, political science, and the social sciences as critical. Hadley and Dooley were both more orthodox and saw psychoanalysis as the organizing discipline. The courses they taught reflected their theoretical leanings. Hadley taught a course on dreams, where the patient's dream became the focus of the work. Sullivan objected to the course. He felt the patient and doctor could get caught in an "obsessional interaction" as they analyzed what the dream meant thereby avoiding other more important material. For Sullivan, dream life was important. The dream was more a signal of something that was happening than a symbol, for example, of "oedipal urges." Unlike his colleagues, Sullivan made use of his dreams as well as those of the patient (Perry, 1982).

Despite these tensions, the Washington School, which was sponsored by the Foundation evolved, with congratulations on its formation from Erich Fromm to Harry Stack Sullivan on October 27, 1939:

> May I express my congratulations [on] your plans. The school promises to become a new beginning and a center of a psychiatry and of psychoanalytic theory, freed from the shackles of sterile dogmatism and fertile through being rooted in the soil of an understanding of culture and social dynamics.

The Foundation led to the incorporation of the William Alanson White Institute of Psychiatry in 1939. Along the way, Clara Thompson was a participant and observer. While she was in Baltimore during the years following her psychiatric training, she had joined the group in its discussions and plans during the fall and winter seasons. She was away in Budapest during the summers. We can only assume she kept in touch with Sullivan about what was transpiring. No correspondence between them covering this period has thus far been found, but we know they were both great letter writers. On her return from Budapest in 1933, she picked up with the activities.

Hale (1995) indicates that in 1939, Lawrence Kubie, then President of the New York Psychoanalytic Society and a member of the new generation, wrote to Glover (who had been his analyst in England) that cliques threatened to destroy the Society:

> Each group is more or less hermetically sealed from the other, and you can imagine how much confusion, lopsided and inadequate training, and mutual distrust and hostility all of this generated.
>
> (p. 141)

Hale recaps the viewpoint that these sealed-up groups fostered animosity against the other groups. Eisold (1998) reiterates Hale's position,

> I believe: the group that coalesced around Horney, outspokenly revisionist, the group around Rado, critical of orthodoxy and seeking ties with medical psychiatry, and the growing group of refugee analysts who had recently fled Hitler. There was, in addition, a small remnant of older members. Finally, there was the group of "young turks," led by Kubie, dedicated to establishing firm and strict standards of training, such as they had themselves experienced abroad.
>
> (Eisold, p. 872)

Shapiro (2017) suggests that Freud's death in 1939, together with the aftermath of the Second World War left the future of psychoanalysis in a state of uncertainty, with people looking for harbors of safety as well as structure. Many European analysts immigrated to America with the hope of restarting their careers and practices.

The Years of Overlap: The New York Psychoanalytic Society (NYPS) and the American Psychoanalytic Association

The New York Psychoanalytic Society was founded in 1911, the same year as the American Psychoanalytic Association. New York Psychoanalytic was a separate organization, but it had overlapping membership with the American Psychoanalytic, which had members from all over the country. The American was comprised of members who were both psychoanalysts and persons interested in psychoanalysis. Adolph Meyer and William Alanson White were charter members of the American, but neither were considered analysts (Thompson, 2017).

The Winds of Change

Thompson recalls that it was Karen Horney who persuaded her to leave the Washington-Baltimore Society and join the New York Psychoanalytic Society. Thompson (2017) said she "was able to endure the New York Society because Horney was in it" (p. 20). They each taught courses and continued to teach at the Washington-Baltimore Institute. In the 1940–1941 catalog of NYPS, Thompson is listed as teaching a course with Lawrence Kubie, whom she would have known from their training at Hopkins under Adolf Meyer. Thompson transferred her membership from Washington-Baltimore to New York and became a member of the New York Psychoanalytic on February 25, 1936. The following November, she was appointed a training analyst. Dr. Nellie Thompson, archivist for NYPS, reports that between May 1937 and December 21, 1937, Thompson didn't attend any meetings of the Society. Shapiro (2017) suggests that there might have been concerns at NYPS about Thompson's reputation based on her having been "chastised" during her training in Baltimore due to rumors about her relationship with her analyst, Joseph Thompson, and because Ferenczi was considered at that point a "heretic by the psychoanalytic establishment" (p. 56). More likely, this was the year Clara Thompson met Henry Major and began a romantic relationship that may have taken more of her time.

In March 1938, she presented a paper to the society (this is listed on the register of her activities in the NYP Society). The Society register indicates that she participated in the discussion of several papers presented at scientific meetings as well as presenting two papers herself (personal communication, Nellie Thompson, September 9, 2020).

Thompson (2017) reports that "Horney was very popular with students" and that her book *The Neurotic Personality of Our Time* stirred-up "a landslide of anger" at New York Psychoanalytic with attempts to isolate Horney:

> So, the New York Psychoanalytic started its system of getting people out of power. The first thing that happened was that her students never graduated. They just never passed the tests. They presented cases, and the teachers said, "Well, that's not psychoanalysis you are doing." So, if you presented a case, and you happened to say something Horney had said, or if it sounded anything like her, the you were not "doing psychoanalysis." This made the students more and more angry, so they began to be rebellious. The next step was to take away Horney's status

as a training analyst, and to demote her to what they called a "lecturer." That is, she was permitted to talk her ideas, but she might not supervise, and she might not analyze students. At the same time, [Abram] Kardiner was getting in bad repute, and his students were having the same kind of trouble. Then mine began to be afraid, too. Although, as usual, I was a little less belligerent than either Kardiner or Horney. But, they caught up with me. So, when they took away Horney's training analyst status, five of us resigned from the New York Psychoanalytic.

(p. 21)

The child psychoanalyst David Levy, a President of the American Psychoanalytic Association, advised the New York Psychoanalytic Institute that an investigation be initiated by the Educational Committee concerning negative feelings among candidates. They declined. Levy took it upon himself to investigate, sending questionnaires out to all the candidates. On April 14, 1941, Levy wrote an unofficial summary of his investigation. He found that students felt, "an unhealthy atmosphere at the Institute due to feelings that within the faculty there are bitter rivalries rancor, dissension, intolerant attitudes an atmosphere of intimidation, etc" (p. 2). The phrases used were taken directly from the replies given in the questionnaire.

There is such an atmosphere of tension in the student body that it is impossible not to be influenced by it. . . . I did not register for a number of courses "for the reason that they were all being conducted by faculty members whose extreme Freudian orthodoxy promised a biased fare to which I had already been too unpleasantly subjected as a Junior student. While I have the highest regard for Freud's genius, I feel at the Institute a not too subtle hostility and contempt for any analyst who attempts to contribute to, modify or contradict on scientific grounds any of the Master's theses.

(Levy letter, p. 2)

On March 26, 1941, Thompson wrote a detailed report[9] about her meeting with the Educational Committee of the New York Psychoanalytic Society, listing her own objections:

I wish to object to the report . . . on the grounds that it is an incomplete statement and by its incompleteness gives an inaccurate impression of my attitude. My real reaction to the interview was that there was no sincere desire on the part of the Educational committee to try to understand my point of view and to rectify misunderstandings. I went away with the impression that their chief concern was to see that their skirts were kept clean. I have this impression on two things: First, the formalistic, lawyer-like way in which my statements were treated. The letter of accuracy of my statements was the concern of the Committee throughout the interview more than the spirit of what I had to say.

The second reason for this impression is . . . many of the statements which I made were thrown out on the technicality that they were second-hand information, being statements made to me by my own students, whose honesty I can personally vouch for. The committee said that since this was second-hand information they did not know that it had happened and therefore could not act on it.

In discussing Topic I of my complaints, they said the following: Concerning the letter they assured me individually that there has been no discussion in the committee, and considering my teaching, as to any non-conservativism being a drawback; that the matter was not mentioned and that the feeling of the committee had been that they were giving me a vote of confidence in asking me to organize the new material in the second half of the course. In response to the statements, I declared that I was satisfied that my non-conservatism was not discussed . . . the educational committee has reported as my saying I was disabused of the impression that the committee intended to discriminate against me. Since the strict accuracy of the statement is being considered, I do not believe that my statement implies as much as the educational Committee has assumed. Moreover, Dr. Zilboorg denied having made the statements to me which I reported. The committee therefore said that he could not take no action on these remarks since it was a question of my word versus Dr. Zilboorg's word, and my memory versus his. Naturally I am not satisfied with this legally correct attitude since I still know that Dr. Zilboorg made these statements. If the Committee had been willing to concede that such things might have been said to me they would have had to concede that at least one person on the committee, i.e. Dr. Zilboorg, had entertained thoughts about my non-conservatism.

In only one of the examples, the first one, did I have the permission of the student to give his name. I did this. Dr. Zilboorg pointed out to the Committee that this student was not a regular student but being analyzed on trial, and naturally tended to have hard feelings about things. This sounded strange to me since no one had ever informed me that he was on trial. Dr. Zilboorg further said that he had personally interviewed him. I have checked up these facts with the student since then and find that he is a fully authorized student and has in his possession a letter to that effect; that he has never at any time been interviewed by Dr. Zilboorg. Obviously, Dr. Zilboorg has confused him with another person, but I wish to point out that his confusion was very convenient at this time.

Concerning Point 2, Dr. Zilboorg felt he may have said some such thing about me in a group and my student happened to be present; that he had not meant it in relation to my educational views, but only politically. My student assures me that it was not said in a group, but to him alone, and that what Dr. Zilboorg meant by it was at least open to question.

As I said in the beginning, the Committee felt nothing could be done about these statements since they were second-hand evidence. The interest of the Committee seemed to be solely concerned with proving that anyway these are not true cases of intimidation, since actually no one has been intimidated as a result. I agreed that in the strict sense of the word no one has been intimidated, but that surely something rotten is going on as evidenced by this.

The Split From New York Psychoanalytic: The Protest

On April 29, 1941, the New York Psychoanalytic Society voted 24 to 7 (with 29 abstentions[10]) to demote Karen Horney's status as training analyst.[11] This rupture culminated in a dramatic moment when Karen Horney with Clara Thompson and others left New York Psychoanalytic:

In dead silence, Karen rose, and with great dignity, her head high, slowly walked out. Thereupon, Thompson, Robbins,[12] Ephron[13] and Sarah Kelman[14] rose and followed her out. They all went to a bar for a few drinks. And then they marched jubilantly down the street, arm in arm, following Thompson's lead in singing Karen's favorite spiritual: "Go down Moses, Way down in Egypt land, Tell old Pharaoh, to let my people go"—the song celebrating the liberation of the Jews from Egyptian tyranny.

(Rubins, 1978, p. 240)

Thompson (2017) clarifies:

> With us went fourteen students; those were my students, Horney's students and Kardiner's students. But Kardiner didn't go with us only his students. As you know, the famous saying is that his students have the courage of his convictions. Silverberg then joined with the five of us and Fromm. And this was the beginning of the Society for the Advancement of Psychoanalysis and the American Institute for Psychoanalysis. This was the Horney group.
>
> (p. 21)

On May 1, 1941, Thompson's formal letter of resignation was delivered:

> My dear Dr. Atkin,
>
> Under the present conditions, I am unwilling to continue teaching my course and have so informed the class. Since my ideas are also undoubtedly suspect, I am sure that this decision will meet with the approval of the Educational Committee.
>
> There should be four more seminars. The reading for next week has been assigned and is the first seven chapters in "The Problem of Anxiety." I had planned to discuss "Civilization and Its Discontents" the following week, and to devote the last two sessions to Anna Freud's book. I mention this simply to give you some idea of the type of material not yet discussed.
>
> I am sure you will have no difficulty in finding someone to complete the course. I shall send in an evaluation of students in due time.
>
> Sincerely yours,
> Clara Thompson, MD

Thompson was done. She knew that only a classical approach to psychoanalysis would be tolerated by the Institute. The final withdrawal from the Institute was followed with a signed formal letter:[15]

> Dear Colleagues:
>
> When five individuals, all teachers of a professional society, feel impelled, for reasons not of a personal nature, to resign their membership in that society, an explanation to their professional colleagues is an obligation upon them and a matter of fundamental importance

to those interested in the profession. The resignations are a response to a situation that constitutes a crisis in psychoanalytic education. Psychoanalysis is a young science, still in an experimental stage of its development, full of uncertainties, full of problems to which anything approaching final and conclusive answers is still to be sought. As in all Sciences, the solutions of these problems are directly dependent upon more voluminous and keener observations, as well as upon further weighing and consideration of observations already made. Education in any field consists in a passing on from an older to a younger generation of the truth that the older generation believes it has learned, as well as it bequeathing to the younger generation the problems left unresolved by their elders. In psychoanalysis as it is today, we cannot afford to subject the younger generation to any dogmatism, we should not miss lead it with the illusion of certainty, where none actually exists. They were two antithetical attitudes towards psychoanalysis today. One of those is based upon the awareness that psychoanalysis is still in an experimental stage of its development. The other attitude regards psychoanalysis as having in many respects past beyond this stage and holds that training and psychoanalysis should begin with the learning of certain concepts and techniques which are, as they sometimes term it, classical, and which represents psychoanalysis as they conceive it to have been 100 handed down by Freud. No two of these classicists have precisely the same notions of what classical psychoanalysis is. But they seem to be agreed that something which passes under the name of classical psychoanalysis should be first inculcated in the student; And that after this certain deviating notions of psychoanalysis may be taught to the student, if he so elects. The educational program which is based upon the conviction that psychoanalytic therapy and therefore theory is still in an experimental stage, and which for want of a better term might be called non-classical is considerably less crystalized than the classical one. It's at its advocates hold that the student at the beginning of his training in psychoanalysis may choose whether he will first be exposed to the classical or to the deviating or non-classical classical concepts. They likewise hold that the student who elects to be personally analyzed by a non-classicist should be taught classical concepts in the course of his training and that the student who chooses a classical type of personal analysis should learn deviating notions as part of his later training. Thus while the classes are very positive about what the beginning of psychoanalytic training should be and are willing to enforce this view where they have the power to do so as in the case of the disqualification of Dr. Karen Horney as a training analyst of the New York Psychoanalytic Institute the non-classics realizing that any crystallization of this nature in the present circumstances premature, are of the opinion that the decision should in each case be left to the individual student. There can be no doubt that there is here drawn a real issue in psychoanalytic education. The issue is, shall policy in the psychoanalytic training be decided upon the basis of the number of votes that can be mustered in favor of this or that theory, or shall we frankly debate I mean admit that it is much too early to attempt a definitive decision of policy? There is no question in the minds of the undersigned that to choose the first of these alternatives will delay rather than accelerate progress, not only in psychoanalytic education but in psychoanalysis itself. Scientific issues cannot be decided by votes or by political power in any form; One would have thought that the experience of Galileo with the church had determined this truth once and for all. We have tried for many years now to come back to this dogmatic dogmatism in psychoanalytic education. Our efforts have increasingly met with frustration; The classicists within the New York psychoanalytic society and his educational committee have become more and more strongly entrenched in their dogmatism, and recent developments have convinced us of the impossibility of persuading them to take a more liberal attitude toward this issue. We have therefore felt it essential for the future of psychoanalysis and psychoanalytic education to dissociate ourselves from a professional organization a majority of whose members are under the impression that scientific issues may legitimately be decided through the possession of political power, and create a new Center for cycle analytic work, devoted to truly liberal and scientific principles, in psychoanalytic training, investigation and discussion period we invite freely all those of our colleagues who are likewise devoted to such principles to join with us in this endeavor.

Signed

Harman Efron, Sarah Kelman, Karen Horney, Bernard Robbins, Clara Thompson

The Association for the Advancement of Psychoanalysis

The day after the walkout from New York Psychoanalytic, the Association for the Advancement of Psychoanalysis was officially organized by the dissenting group, including Horney, Silverberg, Thompson, and others. Fromm and Sullivan became honorary members, while Sullivan maintained his association with the Washington-Baltimore group. According to Perry (1982), the group had been fermenting for some time since "independent thinking of any kind had become increasingly dangerous" (p. 386). Horney was chosen as dean of the Training Institute connected with the new association. But very soon after, divisions developed. Perry suggests that the personal successes of and competitions between Horney and Fromm, combined with the break-up of their long-term romantic relationship, led to bitterness between them. Further, their resentments spilled over into the rest of the psychoanalytic community and were rationalized as theoretical differences about the correct interpretation of Freud's theories:

> Clara Thompson and others, including Sullivan, saw these theoretical differences as a red herring used to disguise more ambitious plans for influence and status. . . . Karen Horney, finally opted for power, deciding that Erich Fromm, her former admired colleague and the person she had recommended as a training analyst for her daughter, would have to be read out of her organization because he did not have a medical degree.
>
> (p. 355)

Another area of contention developed around whether members of the American Psychoanalytic Association who were also members of the new Association for the Advancement of Psychoanalysis in New York would be asked to make a choice of membership. Thompson (2017) provides a clear explanation of the issue:

> The funny thing about this new Society was that it was very much like the Allies in World War II. We were all against the same enemy, but we were not all the same thing. In other words, there were three different ideologies in this group that are symbolized by Kardiner, myself, and Horney, and in our students. But we were starting out with high hopes.

We were going to be open-minded. You could teach anything; you could say anything; and the students were to be encouraged to learn the point of view of everybody. Silverberg was closest to Kardiner's group, I think, so we might group him with them, whereas mine was more in the middle, halfway between the more orthodox orientation and Horney's. In fact, I had never thought of myself as orthodox, but Horney soon seemed to relegate me to that fate, because I found to my horror that a student she sent me, after two or three sessions for supervision, said how disappointed she was because she had come to me to learn the orthodox technique, and Horney had told her that's what I had. Well, I was sorry I couldn't favor her, but. . . . The situation was the Horney group had the most power in that the Society was really formed to protect her. She was the first Dean of this new group, and something began to happen, which of course nobody was responsible for. Presently, it became apparent that no new students were being sent to either Fromm or me.

(p. 23)

The Horney Debacle

Next was a tumultuous break with The Association for the Advancement of Psychoanalysis and with Karen Horney. It evolved sometime around 1943, when tensions between Horney and Fromm flared. Rubin (1978) suggests

the previously submerged interpersonal strains began to surface. Precisely who and what were responsible, whether the differences were ideological or personal, is difficult to pin down. As is to be expected, each of the persons involved has given his own version.

(p. 259)

Sullivan appears to have stayed silent during these tensions. It seems he was hoping a new institute would form that was less conventional. Shapiro (2017) maintains that there was a pressure to "appear respectable in the postwar years when psychoanalysis was establishing its place in American society" (p. 59). That pressure resulted in a conservative environment that, as Shapiro notes, "led to a concern with secrecy and a focus on appearing to be 'normal'" (p. 59). In the mid-1940s legitimacy was a concern. The cohort of European analysts who immigrated during the war years fought to establish their seniority in American psychoanalysis.

The Washington School of Psychiatry in New York

Following the break with Horney, Clara Thompson, Harry Stack Sullivan, Erich Fromm, Frieda Fromm-Reichmann, and colleagues Janet and David Rioch formed the New York Division of the Washington School of Psychiatry. Thompson (2017) provides her own explanation for the relationship between the Washington School of Psychiatry in New York and the Washington-Baltimore Institute:

> So then we met and formed the Washington School of Psychiatry. This happened in 1943 in the spring. . . . There were three people from Washington, and there were Janet [Rioch], Erich [Fromm], and I who were holding the fort up here. So, we had an arrangement: Each one of us went down there every three weeks, rotating, to teach a course in Washington, and Sullivan, Fromm-Reichmann, and David Rioch did the same thing for us; that is, they came up here [New York] in rotating order every three weeks and taught courses here. And this is how the School started.
>
> (p. 23)

As Thompson (2017) explains, and a reading of the history confirms,

> It is very difficult to get clear to you the difference between the Washington School of Psychiatry and the Washington-Baltimore Institute, because in those years, there was no difference. That is, the Washington-Baltimore Institute, was its name when it dealt with the American Psychoanalytic, and the Washington School of Psychiatry was its name when it taught. The reason was that the Washington School of Psychiatry had not been accepted by the American Psychoanalytic when it applied several years before, and had been rejected on the technical basis that it called itself a "school of psychiatry," and therefore, had no place in a psychoanalytic association. So, actually everybody who was in our Institute belonged to two organizations; they belonged the Washington School of Psychiatry and the Washington-Baltimore Institute. I then rejoined the Washington-Baltimore Society, having been without a home for a while, and got back into the American.
>
> (p. 22)

Thompson renewed her membership in the American Psychoanalytic Association and rejoined the Washington-Baltimore Society, but those affiliations soon became problematic. Within six years, around the year of Sullivan's death in 1949, the official tie with Washington was broken, but the unofficial tie continued.

Thompson's first attempt to review the history of William Alanson White Institute of Psychiatry occurred in 1948 as a presentation, modestly titled "Introductory Remarks":

The Birth of the William Alanson White Institute

> Tonight the William Alanson White Institute of Psychiatry holds its first public lecture as an independent institute.
>
> In December 1933, largely at the instigation of Dr. Sullivan, seconded and approved by Dr. White, the William Alanson White Psychiatric Foundation was incorporated in Washington. Its aim was to bring psychiatry in the social sciences together for the purpose of research into the human personality. To accomplish this Dr. Sullivan recommended that psychiatrists should be given the opportunity to profit by the work of the social sciences, and in turn the social sciences should be enriched by education in psychiatric principles.
>
> To further the rapprochement of the two groups, the Washington School of Psychiatry was established in 1936 as a project of the William Alanson White Foundation. For several years the school functioned only in Washington. However, in May 1943, under wartime needs and an increased demand for psychiatric training from members of various professions, it was decided to enlarge the scope of the School and to establish a division in New York City.
>
> The New York Division rapidly increased in size, and in 1946, in order to become chartered under the Board of Regents of the State of New York, a separate corporation was formed which took for its name the William Alanson White Institute of Psychiatry. Under this name, we have held a charter as an educational institution since October 1946.
>
> Although we have changed our name, in most important respects we have not essentially changed our relation to the Washington School of Psychiatry. We are still closely connected in our teaching staff, program, interests, and aims.
>
> Our Institute at the present time offers two types of graduate training. We offer comprehensive training to psychiatrists in the theory

and practice of psychoanalysis. True to Dr. White's vision, we place special emphasis on the relation of personality problems to culture, and our students have the opportunity to become acquainted with the social sciences.

We also provide psychoanalytic orientation to selected professional workers in allied fields, such as medicine, the social sciences, psychology, social work, teaching and the ministry.

The whole spirit and plan of our school was inspired by the vision and active interest of the late William Alanson White, for many years the head of St. Elizabeths Hospital in Washington, D. C. Under his influence, the hospital became one of the foremost institutions for research in and therapy for mental disorder.

Dr. White was a pioneer in modern psychiatry. He, with Brill and Jelliffe, were the first Americans to take an active interest in the then new science of psychoanalysis in the early years of this century.

For many years he and Dr. Jelliffe published the *Psychoanalytic Review*, the first and for a long time the only American psychoanalytic publication. He was a vigorous writer and teacher an open-minded searcher for truth.

Dr. Sullivan and I both had the fortunate experience of working under Dr. White's direction at St. Elizabeth's Hospital around 1920. I am sure Dr. Sullivan will agree with me that he had the quality, all too rare in great thinkers, of inspiring and appreciating the development of those working with him. His interests were not merely limited to hospital problems. He saw psychiatry as having a role to play in the social order, a role greater than the mere care for the mentally ill. He felt the social sciences should collaborate with medicine in seeking the causes of mental disorder in society. To this end he himself was especially interested in the study of crime. In addition to all this, Dr. White was a warm person with many of the traits usually attributed to the old-fashioned general practitioner—that is, a broad human sympathy and a genuine liking for people.

So we are proud to have our Institute bear the name of this pioneer psychiatrist. The roots of our work are in his thinking, and we believe our aims and goals are extensions and outgrowths of his own.

In presenting our Institute for the first time officially to the public, we have chosen as our speaker Dr. Harry Stack Sullivan, the founder of the William Alanson White Foundation, a friend and collaborator of

Dr. White. Dr. Sullivan, whose researches in schizophrenia and whose book *Conceptions of Modern Psychiatry* are well known to many of you, will speak tonight on "The Meaning of Anxiety in Psychiatry and in Life."

Thompson's brief description begins in 1933. While her account is personal and informative, for those seeking more detail, Frosch (1991) presents a broader cast of players and ruptures during these early organizational years. His narrative in particular gives a good description of Horney's dispute with the orthodoxy of New York Psychoanalytic.

In 1937 there was a conflict about a course [Karen Horney] wanted to give which was also given by Rado; she was told her course was unacceptable. At about this time she published *The Neurotic Personality of Our Time* (1937c) which subjected her to many criticisms by more classical analysts. Many felt that the book was essentially directed to a lay public with an emphasis on social factors in psychic development and a deemphasis on childhood factors.

(p. 1044)

In January 1941 Horney was changed from instructor to lecturer. During this time, training analysts were called instructors, and appointed for three-year terms.[16] On April 29 she got up and walked out. Joining her in the walkout were Clara Thompson, Saul Ephron, Bernard Robbins, Sarah Kelman, Janet Rioch, Frances Arkin, Meyer Maskin, Irving Bieber, Sydney Tarachow, George Goldman, Judd Marmor, among others. Rado and Kardiner did not join although many of their students did. . . . The Horney group organized the Association for the Advancement of Psychoanalysis, and a new institute, the American Institute of Psychoanalysis. Sullivan and Erich Fromm joined Ernst Hadley and Benjamin Weininger from the Washington group and N. Lionel Blitsten from Chicago, as well as Stephen Jewett, Chairman of Flower Fifth Avenue Medical School . . . the Association for the Advancement of Psychoanalysis accused the New York Psychoanalytic of misrepresenting them to the New York State Education Department, of not having received a charter as a teaching institute. They threatened to take legal action for what they considered as libel, against the New York, for what they felt was a misrepresentation. There seemed to have been some confusion because there were two legal bodies to grant charters. This was clarified by the two societies, and corrections were made.

Factions seemed to have developed almost from the start in the split-off groups. Horney apparently began to be distressed by Erich Fromm's great popularity with the students of the new institute, and suddenly raised the issue of the inadvisability of having a nonmedical person as a training analyst, although initially she had been quite enthusiastic about the addition of Fromm to the faculty. The raising of this issue seemed designed specifically to push Fromm out of his position of newly acquired prominence in the Institute, and stirred up an enormous amount of bitterness, particularly among Thompson, Sullivan, and their followers. There was a polarization of two groups, one around Horney, and one around Fromm and Thompson. The Horney group had more power, and Thompson and Fromm felt increasingly discriminated against. Another view was opened by retrospective remarks made by Janet Rioch, which placed Sullivan in the background of these events.

There was growing concern that the Association seemed to be becoming a "Horney Group." Thompson and Fromm were angered that most of the new students were taken into analysis by Horney. Horney, in turn, according to several students, appeared to resent Fromm's popularity with students.

Sullivan had been hoping to establish a branch of his Washington School of Psychiatry in New York. Rioch suspected that he subtly promoted the split because he wanted to draw off Thompson and Fromm to form the nucleus of a new group.

Horney and her followers succeeded in voting Fromm out as a training analyst (an ironic duplication of Horney's own previous experience). Thompson, Fromm, Sullivan, and Rioch, together with their students and friends, withdrew from the Association and ultimately, in 1942–1943, formed what is now known as the William Alanson White Institute.

(pp. 1048–1049)

Another historical view that covers this period was delivered by Janet MacKenie Rioch (1959), who focuses on Clara Thompson both before she became the director at WAW and after:

Clara loved her work. Over the years she brought to it a zest and energy and a sort of wide-eyed interest that was unfailing . . . soon after Clara returned to from Budapest to Baltimore, she made another important change in her life—she moved to New York. Here she established her home and practice. She did not, however, lose touch with her Baltimore and Washington associations. She would often go down, in those early years, to the meetings of the Washington-Baltimore Psychoanalytic Society in the good company of Dr. Sullivan and sometimes of Dr. Silverberg and Dr. Horney. . . . These next years were exciting times in the history of psychoanalysis. It was a period of questing and questioning, a period of revolutionary ideas and intellectual ferment and of marked productivity; and Clara was an active and eager part of it. I recall meetings in Washington or Baltimore where Clara and others such as Karen Horney Frida Fromm Reichmann, Erich Fromm, Harry Stack Sullivan and Billy Silverberg took part in stimulating discussions . . .

In the four years during this early New York period, Clara was a training analyst and instructor at the New York Psychoanalytic Institute (1936–1940). She was also Assistant Clinical Professor of Psychiatry at the New York Medical College for three years beginning in 1941. Her close professional associates were Dr. Harry Stack Sullivan and most particularly, Dr. Erich Fromm.

The Washington School of Psychiatry had been established in 1936 as a project of the William Alanson White Foundation. I will read you Clara's own statement about the further developments. "For several years the School functioned only in Washington. However, in May 1943 under pressure of wartime needs and an increased demand for psychiatric training from members of various professions, it was decided to enlarge the scope of the School and to establish a division in New York City." Clara, a natural leader, became head of the New York Division. This was a collaborative venture in which Sullivan and Frieda Fromm-Reichmann came to New York for lectures, seminars and supervision and Clara and I went to Washington to teach and supervise. Clara was a Fellow and faculty member of the School in Washington from 1943 and continued to teach there regularly through 1956.

(pp. 3–6)

Rioch's (1959) history includes the establishment of William Alanson White and Thompson's role in its evolution.

In order to be incorporated under the New York State Board of Regents, the New York division of the Washington School formed a separate corporation 1946 and took for its name the William Allison White Institute of Psychiatry. In 1951 it received a permanent charter as the William Allison White Institute of Psychiatry, Psychoanalysis and Psychology. Clara became the executive director and president of the board of trustees and remained in these positions until the time of her death. All during this time without any interruption since 1943 Clara taught courses and seminars. In addition to being the director and attending practically all of the meetings connected with the school and going to many of the courses . . . the above activities constituted only a small portion of Clara's active professional life. She spent most of her time 9 to 10 hours a day, five to six days a week in doing therapy and supervision she loved the work and she read or rejoiced in the flourishing of the Institute. Clara was very much interested in the training of students from other countries and also was actively helpful in arranging to overcome the technical and practical problems involved. She was especially interested in the development of the Institute of Psychiatry founded in Brazil by one of our graduates, the late doctor Tracy Doyle. At Dr. Doyle's invitation Clara went to Rio de Janeiro the summer of 1955 to teach and give a seminar. She enthusiastically encouraged others to do the same thing in the following summers.

(p. 6)

Rioch also adds to our understanding of an important dimension of Thompson's personality: "She was always trying to get to the heart of things and always trying to make sense" (p. 6).

Trying to make sense—and get to the heart of things—certainly kept Thompson engaged and in each of these organizations. While at the same time she was developing a model of therapy that emphasized the continuous co-participation and mutual influence of the patient and analyst. This brand of psychoanalysis was associated with WAW and is known as interpersonal psychoanalysis.

Notes

1 A short two-page, the history of the Washington Psychoanalytic Society is available at Washington Psychoanalytic Society Encyclopedia.com. It is drawn from, Noble, Douglas, and Burnham, Donald. (1969). *History of the Washington Psychoanalytic Society and the Washington Psychoanalytic Institute*. Washington DC: Washington Psychoanalytic Society.

2 Studies in Hysteria by Freud and Breuer was published as a paper in 1893 and the book in 1895.

3 See Rand B. Evans and William A. Koelsch's (1985) Psychoanalysis Arrives in America: The 1909 Psychology Conference at Clark University. *American Psychologist.* 40(8), 942–948.

4 Freud considered an international organization to be essential to the promotion of his ideas and in 1910, the International Psychoanalytic Association (IPA) was established with Carl Jung as president.

5 With the First World War, the field of psychiatry developed a new sense of mission and an expanded role. For example, *Freud's (1915) Reflections on War and Death* painted a grim picture of the human race; in contrast, William Alanson White (1919) wrote *Thoughts of Psychiatrists on the War and After* with a less darker perspective. In White's view was a version of 'if it does not kill you it makes you stronger,' or, over-coming obstacles can be a positive influence in the development of character. (Hale, 1995, p. 23)

6 Sandor Rado, a Hungarian psychoanalyst who moved the United States in the 1930s.

7 In Chicago, in 1932, the Institute for Psychoanalysis was founded by Franz Alexander, which consisted of notable psychoanalysts, including Karen Horney, among others.

8 Polly Adler survived by paying half of her income to underworld mobsters like Dutch Schultz. Her best-selling book *A House Is Not a Home* (1953) was adapted into film by the same name.

9 Discussion of Report of Educational Committee, March 26, 1941. WAW archives.

10 Rubins (1978) explains that the 29 abstentions were either "German-speaking colleagues," who though disagreed with her were still "friendly and sympathized with her" but couldn't bring themselves to reject her, and people who were themselves preparing to leave the society and didn't want to tip their hand. (p. 240).

11 She was allowed to keep candidates already in analysis but not allowed to take new candidates into analysis.

12 Bernard Robbins, MD, one of the founders of the Association for the Advancement of Psychoanalysis.

13 Harmon Ephron, MD, one of the founders of Association of Advancement of Psychoanalysis and the American Institute for Psychoanalysis who co-taught courses with Karen Horney and Erich Fromm at the New School for Social Research. His first analyst was Abraham Kardiner whom he described as "inert"; his second analyst was Karen Horney (Memorial by Leland van den Daele, September 23, 2016).

14 Sarah Kelman, MD, was first a nurse then a physician and a graduate of New York Psychoanalytic Institute and member of William Alanson White Psychoanalytic Society.

15 The letter is signed by Harmon S. Ephron, Sarah R. Kelman, Karen Horney, Bernard S. Robbins, and Clara Thompson. WAW archives.

16 Training analysts needed to be renewed after each three-year term.

References

Adler, P. (1953). *A House Is Not a Home*. Rinehart & Co, New York.

Benveniste, D. (2006). The early history of psychoanalysis in San Francisco. *Psychoanalysis and History*, *8*(2), 195–233.

Bullard, D. (1969). "Talk" by Dr. Dexter Bullard. The Oskar Diethelm library DeWitt Wallace institute for the history of psychiatry. Weill Cornell Medical College Harry Stack Sullivan Series I, 1927–1982, Box 1, Series 1.

Burnham, J. (1956). The beginnings of psychoanalysis in the United States. *American Imago, Spring*, *13*(1), 65–68.

Chapman, A. H. (1976). *Harry Stack Sullivan: His life and his work*. New York: Putnam Adult.

Eisold, K. (1998). The splitting of the New York psychoanalytic society and the construction of psychoanalytic authority. *The International Journal of Psychoanalysis*, *79*, 871–885.

Eisold, K. (2003). The profession of psychoanalysis: Past failures and future possibilities. *Contemporary Psychoanalysis*, *39*(4), 557–582.

Eisold, K. (2018). Psychoanalytic training: Then and now. In P. Zagermann (Ed.), *The future of psychoanalysis: The debate about the training analyst system* (pp. 53–69). London: Routledge.

Evans, R. B., & Koelsch, W. A. (1985). Psychoanalysis arrives in America: The 1909 psychology conference at Clark University. *American Psychologist*, *40*(8), 942–948.

Frosch, J. (1991). The New York psychoanalytic civil war. *Journal of the American Psychoanalytic Association*, *39*(4), 1037–1064.

Funk, R. (2000). *Erich Fromm: His life and ideas*. New York: A&C Black.

Green, M. (1964). Her life. In M. Green (Ed.), *Interpersonal psychoanalysis the selected papers of Clara M. Thompson*. New York and London: Basic Books.

Hale, N. G. (1995). *The rise and crisis of psychoanalysis in the United States*. Oxford: Oxford University Press.

Jones, E. (1934) Letter to A.A. Brill, Archives British Psychoanalytic Society, London, England.

Lionells, M. (2017). Yesterday and Today: Reflections on Clara Thompson's history of the White Institute. *Contemporary Psychoanalysis*, *53*(1), 37–43.

Noble, D., & Burnham, D. (1969). *History of the Washington psychoanalytic society and the Washington psychoanalytic institute*. Washington, DC: Washington Psychoanalytic Society.

Paris, B. (1994). *Karen Horney: A psychoanalyst's search for self-understanding*. Yale University Press, New Haven.

Perry, H. S. (1982). *Psychiatrist of America: The life of Harry Stack Sullivan*. Cambridge, MA: Belknap Press.

Rioch, J. M. (1959). Clara Thompson: Her professional life and work. *The Newsletter of the White Institute*, *7*(1).

Rubins, J. L. (1978). *Karen Horney: Gentle rebel of psychoanalysis*. New York: The Dial Press.

Shapiro, S. A. (2017). The history of the William Alanson White Institute sixty years after Thompson. *Contemporary Psychoanalysis*, *53*(1), 44–62.

Thompson, C. (1948). Introductory remarks. Proceedings on the occasion of the first William Alanson White Memorial Award, WAW Archives.

Thompson, C. (1958). A study of the emotional climate of psychoanalytic institutes. *Psychiatry*, *21*(1), 45–51.

Thompson, C. (2017). The history of the William Alanson White Institute. *Contemporary Psychoanalysis*, *53*(1), 7–28.

Chapter 3

Summers in Provincetown
From Repression to Expression

599 Commercial Street

For Clara Thompson, Provincetown was a place of tranquility and love. She purchased a former sailboat house at 599 Commercial Street in Provincetown, MA. The home offered stunning views of the harbor and a place to watch the ebb and flow of the tides. All her life she enjoyed swimming and the sea. It must have felt like a dream come true. Summers in Provincetown brought a breath of fresh sea air and a feeling of freedom into her life. From 1939 until her death in 1958, she owned this iconic waterfront home. While her time in Provincetown was mostly tranquil, she still had a lot to juggle during her summers: her relationship with Henry Major, the complicated political ground at analytic institutes, her patients, and her clinical scholarship.

Falling in Love: Henry Major

In the spring of 1938, Clara Thompson had gone with a friend to see the work of a new Hungarian artist, Henry Major. They met, fell in love, and began a relationship that lasted nearly a decade. Thompson and Major were devoted to each other. She was 45; Major was 49 and married to Elizabeth Alexander. He had married Alexander in 1924 and they immigrated to the United States in 1927. Little is known about Elizabeth Alexander, except that she was a voice coach. Henrich (Henry) Major, born in Nagyszalonta, Hungary, was a world-famous cartoonist and artist. For a short time, he lived in France before immigrating. He was a self-taught painter and former pupil at the Budapest Academy, where he studied for three months. His obituary notes that he left the Academy because he did not like the ideas they taught (The Provincetown Advocate, 1948). In the

DOI: 10.4324/9781003284840-4

winter, Major lived with his wife Elizabeth in New York, and in the summer he lived with Clara Thompson in Provincetown. Sprague (2001) suggests that Thompson not only accepted the limitations of their relationship but perhaps preferred them.

One can easily imagine these two rebels breaking with conventions and finding love as they comfortably made their home in this community of vacationing analysts, accomplished artists, Portuguese immigrants, renown intellectuals, and writers. They cultivated a Provincetown circle of friendships. Some came to him for painting lessons in the shack Thompson built for Major in her front yard. They enjoyed life, spending their days doing what they loved (D'Ercole, 2017). We don't know how Elizabeth Alexander felt about their arrangement. Perhaps she too was content with it. There is speculation that religious convictions or possibly some illness kept them from divorcing, but we don't know.

Henry Major was known for his caricatures of famous people, including Albert Einstein and others, as well as his artist sketches as he covered the Lindbergh trial for his job at the Hearst papers. As a caricaturist and a keen observer, his perceptions of people would have been appealing to Thompson, and her understanding of character equally appealing to him. Major said that Provincetown reminded him of his birthplace. His Hungarian heritage undoubtedly reminded her of Ferenczi and her time in Budapest.

Peter Manso (2002) colorfully describes the art scene in Provincetown, commencing with the wave of artists who arrived in Provincetown at the end of the 19th century to work with Charles Webster Hawthorne in his Cape Cod School of Art. Hawthorne was an American painter renowned for his lush portraits and landscapes. Manso notes that arriving artists paid as little as $50 a year for studio space. The Provincetown Art Association, formed in 1914, became the site of the struggle between the Hawthorne traditionalists and the modernists. In the early 1930s, modernism made its way to the Outer Cape, including the vibrant paintings of E. Ambrose Webster and the watercolors and paintings of the gay painter, Charles Demuth. The art wars in Provincetown were a turning point in the art scene.

The year before Thompson and Major settled into 599 Commercial Street, the Provincetown Art Association had staged an extraordinary show at its annual exhibition, a compromise between modernists and conventional painters. As the program for the Provincetown Art Association (1938) highlights: "There have come on the scene a number of young artists who view dispassionately what were once burning questions of art dogma." The clash between the old and new guard in the Provincetown art world in ways paralleled what was occurring in the world of psychoanalysis, the struggle between the orthodox and non-Freudian analysts. In art, the dogma of traditional art was being replaced by the modernists; psychoanalytic dogma was being challenged by non-Freudian culturalists promoting new clinical formulations and methods of working.

Psychoanalysis itself was no stranger to Provincetown. A few doors away from Thompson at 621 Commercial Street, the Pulitzer Prize winner Susan Glaspell staged the first production of *Suppressed Desires*, a clever comedy that poked fun at unconscious wishes disguised in dreams, reducing Freud to a game of "you tell me your dreams and I'll tell you mine!" (Ben-Zvi, 2005).

Summering in Provincetown during Thompson's era was affordable. In 1939, a full course meal could be enjoyed for $0.50 at the Atlantic House. For Clara Thompson who loved to dance, their advertisement in the local newspaper welcoming people to the "best dance floor in the center of town" (Provincetown Art Association, 1939) might have been appealing. Dinners and lunches at the Lobster House started at $0.65 cents.

Thompson was in tune with the emergent attitudes of the 1920s, not only in art and psychoanalysis but with the sense of social responsibility and the growing criticism of gender roles and marriage as an institution. Many intellectuals and artists believed marriage would interfere with their creativity.

The artistic scene in Provincetown fit well with both Thompson and Major's unconventional relationship; their rejection of orthodoxy likely nurtured their rebellious spirits. They each resisted being boxed-in or tied to a domineering system. Major had adopted the tag, "the gay philosopher." He sold a wide variety of memorabilia from posters to playing cards that carried his signature characters. For example, I purchase a sturdy red and gold box holding a deck of cards. The inside cover of the box tells the following story,

> Henry Major is internationally famous as a serious painter. But he has his lighter side, and here, in "Ma & Pa Philosopher," he has combined a keen insight into human nature, and a fine sense of humor in masterful portrayal of two citizens of the world. It takes only a moment after the first chuckle to see that the artist has captured his subjects' relaxed disregard for needless hustle and bustle. They know satisfaction in the simple things of life.

>May they bring you moments of pleasant relaxation and the opportunity for reflection on the good things of life.

The image of "Pa" resembles Henry Major. Could "Ma" possibly be Clara Thompson?

The Great Depression and War Years

The changes in the art scene in Provincetown were driven to some degree by the Great Depression. The fishing industry had previously sustained Provincetown. Krahulik (2007) describes how during the second half of the great depression the fishing industry in Provincetown suffered and its economy was rescued by Franklin D. Roosevelt's Works Progress Administration (WPA). The WPA program financially supported Provincetown artists.

Clara Thompson's neighbors, Philip Malicoat, Blanche Lazzell, and George Yater, were among those selected for the Federal Arts Project (FAP) and Federal Theater Project (FTP), which funded paintings, murals, and plays. There was a hierarchy of pay from the WPA, with the FAP recipients receiving higher weekly salaries. This hierarchy created a tension. Earlier lending a hand or a neighborly exchange helped the troubled Provincetown economy; this new source of money created a disparity between those who received greater or lesser amounts of federal help.

John (Ike) Taylor Williams[1] (2022) describes prominent leftists and their political activism in Provincetown. He views Provincetown between 1910 and 1960 as a hotbed of new ideas. No doubt this hotbed of new ideas influenced both art and the psychoanalysts like Clara Thompson who summered there. The "bohemians" who came to the Cape "brought their new acadia easels and typewriters and a distaste for money not earned by creativity; their obsession with alcohol as a muse; their commitment to sexual freedom for both men and women, married and unmarried; and very little interest in their own children, if child-rearing in any way interfered with these pursuits" (Taylor Williams, 2022, p. 15). One of Thompson's neighbors, Mary Heaton Vorse, was a journalist, novelist, and activist. Vorse wrote about the struggles of her generation of American women. Vorse, only a year older than Thompson, was from the same cohort of 20th-century women. Joanna Scutts (2019) points to how they were called "New Women" similar to the "Modern Women" that Thompson addressed in her essays and the views she shared with Karen Horney. One can easily envision these two "modern/new women" sitting on the deck at Thompson's house or in the garden at Vorse's home comparing their experiences and their evolving gender analysis.

During the war years because of Provincetown's location at the most eastern point of the United States, residents feared an invasion could come by way of the shores of the Atlantic. The *Sunday Cape Cod Times* (June 19, 1983) reports that there were rumors of spies landing in Maine and that the greatest scare came when on June 6, 1942, the *SS Cherokee*, a freighter-passenger steamship, was struck by two torpedoes about 62 miles east of Provincetown. The ship traveling from England to New York sank, killing 86 of the 169 aboard. Forty-two survivors were brought to Provincetown. The town pulled together to care for them. Thompson alongside other doctors, first-aid workers, ambulances, and air raid wardens could easily have been one of those who came to their assistance.

For Thompson and Major, summers in Provincetown were a long season that began in June and extended through September.

Thompson and Major spent time with each other in New York City as well, though one can imagine that their meetings were complicated by the presence of Major's wife. Thompson's fall to spring schedule was full, her private practice busy, and leadership of the Institute demanded much of her time. She saw patients daily. Major too was busy with his work at the Hearst papers.

Unexpectedly, Elizabeth Alexander died in a car accident in August 1948. Shortly after the accident, Thompson wrote to her friend Ralph Crowley (Letter to Crowley, August 29, 1948): "So suddenly after all these years we are free." That short note only hints at her feelings. Alexander's death must have elicited many ambivalent feelings, sadness, guilt, relief, and perhaps trepidation about this new freedom. In her letter to Ralph Crowley, we again experience her unvarnished matter-of-fact-ness, a communication style we have come to expect.

In 1947, Henry Major had become ill with lung cancer. Thompson cared for him at the house on Commercial Street. His death in the fall of 1948, at the age of 59 was a devastating blow. His obituary in the Provincetown Advocate notes that he was known all over Provincetown as "the artist who painted on red canvas" and that Erich Fromm, the well-known analyst and author, gave a eulogy (Major, 1948). A painting of his is held in the collection of the Provincetown Art Museum (see photo exhibit).

Thompson was very fond of Major's nephew and "practically adopted him as a foster son" (Green, 1964, p. 371.) She also provided financial support to Hungarian immigrants. A recent finding identified Henry Major's nephew, Nicholas (Miklos) Major, and his wife Eva, among the 1600 Hungarian Jewish refugees aboard the famous Kastner train headed for a death camp (Porter, 2009). Rudolf Kastner, a Jewish Hungarian journalist, negotiated with Adolf Eichmann for the ransom of the sixteen hundred Jews aboard the train. They were safely brought to Switzerland. Anna Porter (2009) describes the rescue and tragic aftermath that led to Kastner's assassination in Israel.

In 1950, Eva and Nicholas divorced. He boarded a ship in France (the Veendam) and made his way to the United States. The ship's registry lists Clara Thompson as the person designated to vouch for and support him. Nicholas (Miklos), is named in Thompson's will. She bequeathed him all of Henry's paintings.

Life Goes On

Following Major's death, Thompson continued to summer in Provincetown. In 1949, Harry Stack Sullivan died delivering another serious loss. In a memorial service on February 11, 1949, Thompson described their relationship:

> Our mutual interest in patients was a very strong bond between us. We early discovered that we both had the same kind of feeling for patients, a genuine liking and respect. His ideas about patients always seemed to make sense to me, and I absorbed them intuitively and almost unconsciously. I soon learned that this man, who in public could tear a bad paper to bits with his scathing sarcasm, had another side—a gentle, warm, friendly one. This was the side he showed to his patients. Anyone who has seen him talking with a disturbed catatonic can know that he has seen the real Harry without pretense or defenses. There was nothing maudlin about his tenderness—it rather conveyed the feeling of deep understanding.
>
> The quality of his friendship showed the same genuineness and tolerance so characteristic of his relation to patients. He was slow in making friends. He tested them for a long time: Were they over-competitive or neurotically ambitious? Did they have jealous natures? Were they

opportunistic? For these characteristics he had no tolerance. Once a person had passed the test he could count on Harry for absolute loyalty. No matter what your mistakes—and he might point them out to you privately—before the world he was on your side. I once had reason to be grateful for this loyalty in a situation where a lesser man might have been concerned with the possible jeopardy to his own status by defending me. I believe that self-interest never had any weight with him when loyalty to a friend was the issue. In all crisis he was at hand.

(Thompson, 1964, pp. 371–372)

Thompson's gratitude to Sullivan for his loyalty likely refers to her clash with Adolf Meyer in Baltimore when Meyer insisted that she stop seeing her then-analyst Joseph Thompson. She subsequently resigned from Meyer's clinic.

Clara Thompson was also grateful to Erich Fromm whom she relied on during these difficult times, but Fromm was having his own troubles. His wife was ill, and he decided in 1949 that Mexico's climate would be best for her. His move there was also a loss for Thompson.

She threw herself into her work to advance the William Alanson White Institute. Green explains that Thompson was "annoyed and impatient with the American Psychoanalytic Association for their four-year period of procrastination concerning the application of the White Institute for full accreditation as a training facility under its aegis" (p. 373).

She was ultimately relieved though disappointed when the approval of the application to the American seemed hopeless, and the decision was made to withdraw it. She turned her attention to organizing the Academy of Psychoanalysis so that the Institute could be part of a wider community. While life was full in Provincetown, work was never far from Thompson's mind.

In 1950, a friend visited her and said:

Clara, as I knew her that summer, was a revelation of how life can be fulfilled. She had so many sides—housewife and cook, with the chores of cleaning left to the capable hands of a Portuguese woman who came in just long enough to do them. She was the hostess with hardly a day going by that some guests other than us weren't entertained. She was a writer, spending every morning at it religiously. And she was an analyst, having two or three regularly scheduled patients and occasionally seeing emergencies. I remember hearing the voices from upstairs from a three-hour session that Clara had with an internationally famous woman who flew to Provincetown for a consultation. The first hour was stormy, high pitched, and continuous; then occasionally Clara's low, gentle murmur; then, in response, a gradual diminuendo; ending in tones barely audible, harmonious, and almost happy. I saw the patient as she left, looking sparkling and poised. Clara seemed a little tired, but not disturbed, and we went on to other afternoon business as usual. We went to lectures and plays in the evening, or visited some friends, sometimes went to an evening party or held one, or just stayed home, talked, and read. It seemed to me that Clara had everything anyone could want to enrich her life— professional achievement, contact with all the activities of the mind, friends, comfort, security (as much as she wanted of it), and freedom. But it wasn't enough.

(Green, 1964, p. 373)

She encouraged patients to come to Provincetown and continue their treatment in the summer; many did. She took long daily swims in the bay and scheduled analytic sessions around them. Sometimes a change was made to a patient's appointment to take advantage of the tide, a custom that led to some confusion for her patients, who were not as attuned to the ebb and flow. Her attitude was relaxed. She was less formal than others in her profession. Green found her to be shy with children but once she got to know them she was "like another child herself" (p. 370). She had frequent parties where alcohol flowed freely. A friend asked her, "Clara, how can you stand it?" meaning all the people, she replied, "You must know by now that I just like people, I just accept them, I don't analyze them" (p. 371). Patients were included in her parties. Ruth Moulton (1969), a psychoanalyst and former analysand of Thompson, recalls how her then supervisor, Harry Stack Sullivan, warned her

against excessive socializing with patients, having seen a good deal of this in Provincetown. He felt that Clara Thompson could get away with seeing many of her patients and students in that casual summer setting but that most students could not afford to do the same with their own patients. In the first place, few possessed Clara's quiet, unanxious simplicity; besides, no student would be able to handle whatever reactions his patients might have to observing the therapist's private life. Sullivan felt that patients would then be apt to withhold reactions that might make the therapist uneasy, thus making it impossible to work through parataxic distortions.

(p. 155)

Sullivan's advice flew past Thompson's ears. She did not heed her own words of warning about the pitfall of socializing with her patients. Her informal "open house" parties were legendary, with the combination of Portuguese fishermen and bohemian artists that mixed comfortably with patients and colleagues. She routinely rode her bike to the market and purchased bread from the Portuguese bakery. She grew her own vegetables, had a flair for Hungarian cooking, and loved to dance. Lillie Fisher, Thompson's housekeeper in New York, accompanied her to Provincetown for the first few summers but did not enjoy the Cape. Perhaps she felt the Cape was too far from her relatives in Baltimore. Thompson employed a local housekeeper, yet she still did her own shopping piling her groceries into the basket on the front of her bicycle. Green (1964) reports that all her neighbors knew her and felt warmly toward her. Her brother Frank and sister-in-law Peg visited with their two young daughters Sue and Frances at the end of each summer, as did various students, patients, and friends.

Thompson grew particularly close to her neighbors Philip and Barbara Malicoat. Philip Malicoat was a well-known painter in Provincetown. He and his wife were a central part of the thriving Provincetown art scene, and Thompson became a part of the Malicoat family. Malicoat built the deck on her house and most of its furniture. There were rumors of a romance between Thompson and Malicoat sometime after Henry Major's death. Whatever the truth it has passed on with them. Upon her death, Clara Thompson left her home on Commercial Street to both Philip and Barbara Malicoat (see last will)—a very generous gift.

Around Town

Although the people I interviewed in town remembered Thompson, there was scant detailed information. If there was a memory to tell, it was always conveyed with warmth and respect, generally revealing the soft and playful side to Thompson. The author Peter Manso, son of the Provincetown painter Leo Manso, happily recalls running into Thompson with her pockets filled with a new litter of kittens. The image conjures up Thompson's love of cats. The year was probably 1956, when Thompson's cat Mochka had just given birth to a litter. Another Commercial Street neighbor, Christopher Busa, son of renowned painter Peter Busa, remembers Thompson as a family friend. Another neighbor recalled only her grey hair, her prominence as a New York psychoanalyst, and whispers of an affair with a neighbor. Anton "Napi" Van Derecks, a local restaurant owner and avid collector of Provincetown artists' works, recalled artists of the era who were in psychoanalytic treatment with major New York analysts. How many were referred to those analysts by Thompson is difficult to know but given the close ties among the community's artists and intellectuals and Thompson's vast referral resources, one can infer it was a significant number. Painter Salvatore Del Deo recalled a famous female psychoanalyst living in Provincetown but did not know Thompson himself. That Thompson was remembered is not surprising; she had a natural capacity for warmth and kindness.

The "Girdle Brigade"

Thompson's humor, warmth, and joie de vie are revealed in an exchange of a set of three beautiful hand-painted watercolor note cards done by Sylvia Smith, an artist and apparent friend of Clara Thompson. The four women, Sylvia, Elsa, Fanny, and Clara must have been in Provincetown together and sent these greetings when Elsa was absent and for her birthday.[2]

In what turned out to be a very fortunate purchase, John Betagole found a copy of Thompson's (1950) *Psychoanalysis Evolution and Development* at a library sale in Cincinnati about 20 years ago. The book with a bookplate by Stanley L. Block is inscribed, "To Elsa, the guardian of my peace with love, Clara." Suggesting the book had been given to Elsa Weihl by Clara Thompson, and later came into the possession of Dr. Block, a prominent Cincinnati psychoanalyst. Elsa Weihl is the co-author of *That Man Heine*, a German poet whose lyrics were set to music by Schubert and Schumann. Weihl may have lived in New Hampshire. I speculate that she might have been a friend of Izette de Forest who lived in New Hampshire too.

In the book was an envelope addressed to Miss Elsa Weihl at the Mt. Crescent House, Randolph Hill, Randolph, New Hampshire with a return address to Thompson in Provincetown. One of the cards dated August 4, 1954, is a birthday greeting. One card, a watercolor painting of Clara Thompson's house includes greetings from Clara Thompson's niece Sue, who would have been 22 at the time, indicating that her niece continued to visit her aunt beyond her visits as a young child with her parents. There is a joyfulness and casual flair in the communication, reflecting the mood of Thompson's time in Provincetown.

Creating hand-painted cards was a practice in Provincetown during that era. The note card dated August 4, 1954, references "girdles." This note card painting is whimsical and features a woman sitting in a rocking chair in her underwear, bra, girdle, garters, and stockings. In the greeting Fanny refers to the "girdle brigade," which apparently consisted of Clara Thompson, Elsa Weihl, Sylvia Smith, and 'Fanny.' Betagole brought these items to the attention of Dr. Peter Rudnytsky, who knew I would be interested in the memorabilia. It is through the generosity of John Betagole and Peter Rudnytsky that we get to view these charming exchanges.

Along with the cards were several newspaper clippings of Thompson's obituary from December 20, 1958, and a clipping of a *New York Times* April 24, 1959, article, "*Position Defined by Neo-Freudian: Fromm rejects role as an anti-Freudian as he cites new gains in knowledge.*" Erich Fromm is quoted as saying,

> there is a marked difference between neo-Freudianism and anti-Freudianism . . . neo- Freudians were not a unified school of psychoanalysts. Rather, he declared they are made up of various groups that share a common objective: to build upon the knowledge of Sigmund Freud and the techniques of psychoanalysis in view of what is known a generation after Freud founded psychoanalysis.

Fromm's remarks were made at the first annual Clara Thompson Memorial Lecture in her honor. He notes that she was "a founder of neo-Freudianism."

Among these clippings was an invitation to the opening of the "Clara Thompson Building at the William Alanson White Institute."

> #1. This watercolor is a beautiful depiction of Thompson's house viewed from the water. It reads,
> August 4, 1954
> Dear Elsa
> 6 kittens born yesterday with a whole school of midwives. Kittens all well & Mochka slinks by . . . we loved your letter—shocked about girdles, anyway here's the house to be with you.
> Love, Clara

Also,

Hello Elsa—

Although we're sorry we sort of dispossessed you, we're appreciating it (the house & all) not only for ourselves but for you too.

P'town & above are Clara & her house is triply wonderful after NY & its weather.

Love, Fanny

And,

Dear Elsa—

Clara kindly allowed us to read your wonderful letter.-"The Rocking chair and the Forbidding Faces" reminded me of one of my earliest vacations spent with my grandmother. After a while, however, "the forbidding faces" became real nice, friendly human beings, and I hope you will have the same good luck.

We are having a glorious time here—and our only complaint is that time speeds by too rapidly. Clara's niece, Sue, joins me in wishing you a happy vacation.

Love, Sylvia

#2. Depicts an iconic view of Provincetown harbor and monument. It reads,

Just thinking about your birthday,

Love, Clara

And,

A very happy birthday to you, Elsa. Every good wish.

Sylvia Smith

#3. Is a painting of a woman in glasses sitting in a rocking chair wearing her bra, girdle, garters and stockings. It reads,

You see the kind of picture you paint of your vacation. Anyway don't

let the Grant Woods spoil your birthday.

Love, Clara

And,

Happy Birthday to Elsa. Hope the girdle brigade don't get too chilled.

Love, Fanny

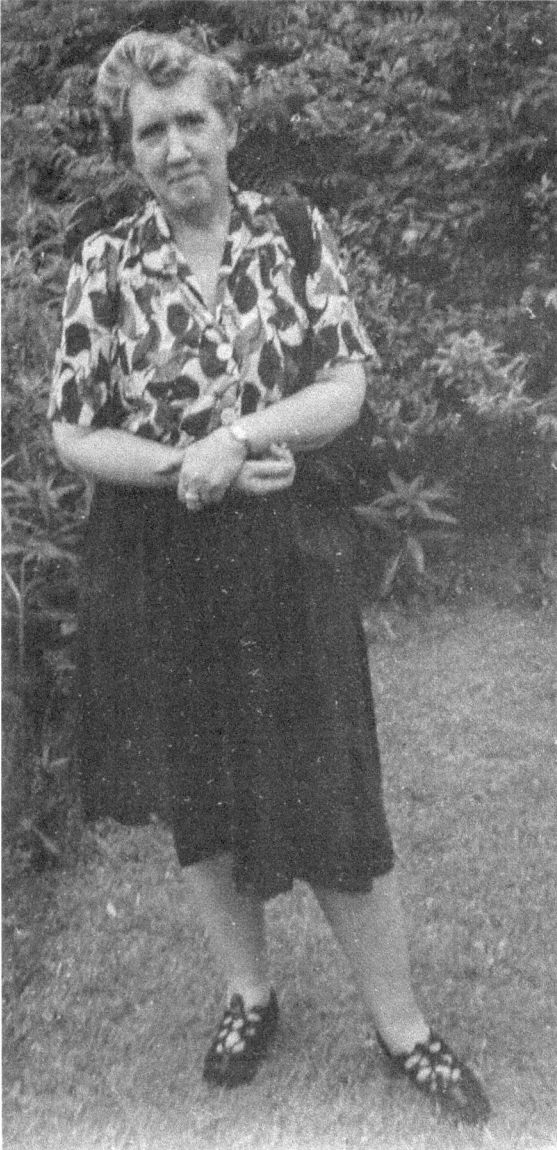

Figure 3.1 Clara Thompson in Provincetown circa 1940. Reprinted with permission, © William Alanson White Institute.

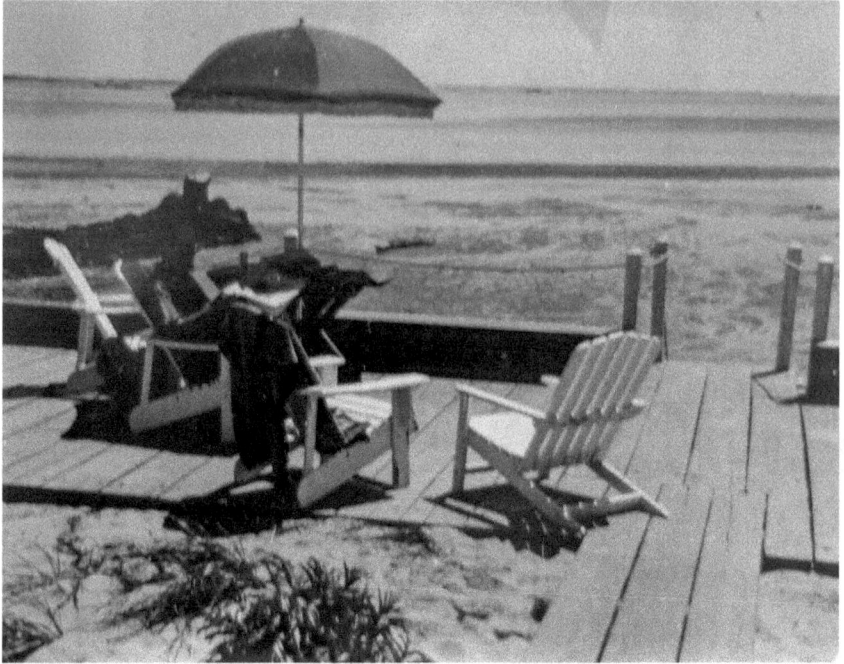

Figure 3.2 Clara Thompson's deck facing the bay. Reprinted with permission, © William Alanson White Institute.

LGBTQ Retreat

Provincetown is a beach lover's paradise in winter or summer. The three-mile-long strip of town was incorporated in 1720. As the writer Michael Cunningham (2002) observes, "On stormy days gusts of sand still blow through the streets" (p. 15). Provincetown's relative geographic isolation has helped to shelter the unconventional seeking a place to feel free from stigma and pressures to conform.

In the early 20th century particularly in the summers, it became home to the LGBTQ+ community. No doubt that the community had some influence on her. During her years in residence in Provincetown, Thompson wrote, "Changing Concepts of Homosexuality in Psychoanalysis" (1947). The paper claims several conflicting ideas, including once you clear up all the other personality issues, homosexuality would go away. Her friendships with Harry Stack Sullivan and his aunt Margaret Stack, James Inscoe, Ruth Benedict, Margaret Mead, Izette de Forest, and Alice Lowell are just a few

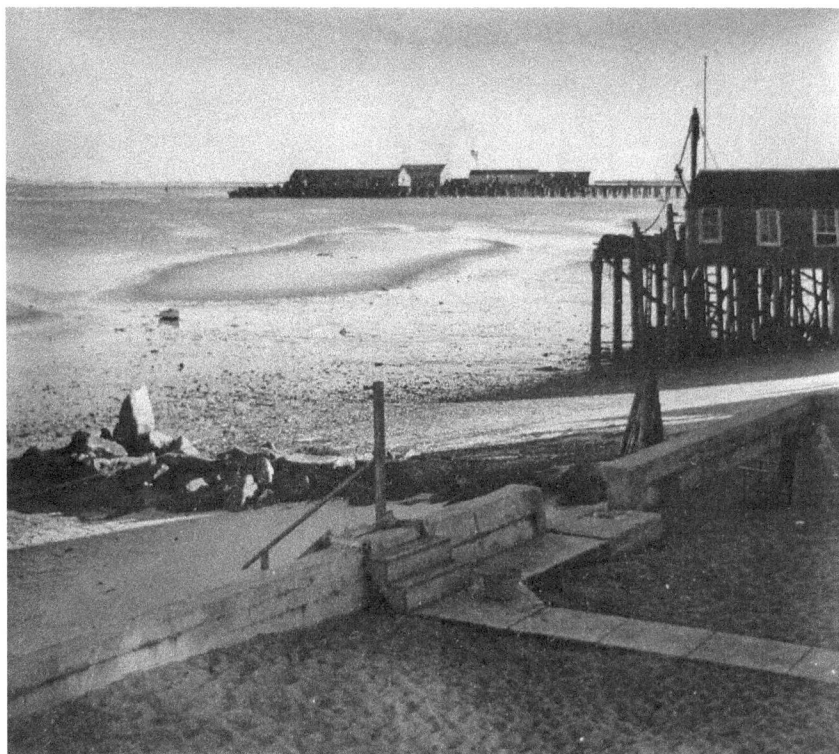

Figure 3.3 View from the deck. Reprinted with permission, © William Alanson White Institute.

of the [sexually] and gender non-conforming people who were part of her social life. They influenced her but did not bring her to more progressive conclusions in her professional writing. She accepted the idea of a homosexual marriage and grappled with the messy psychoanalytic construct of homosexuality, concluding it was too narrowly defined. She noted how when a boy is called a sissy he is stigmatized, and feels belittled, but when a girl is called a tomboy, she feels a sense of pride. She opined:

> Probably the names get their value from childhood ideas that courage and daring are desirable traits in both sexes. So, the sissy is a coward, a mama's boy, and the tomboy, is a brave girl who can hold her own with a boy her size. These attitudes probably became a part of later attitudes toward homosexuality in the two sexes.
>
> (Thompson, 1947, p. 186)

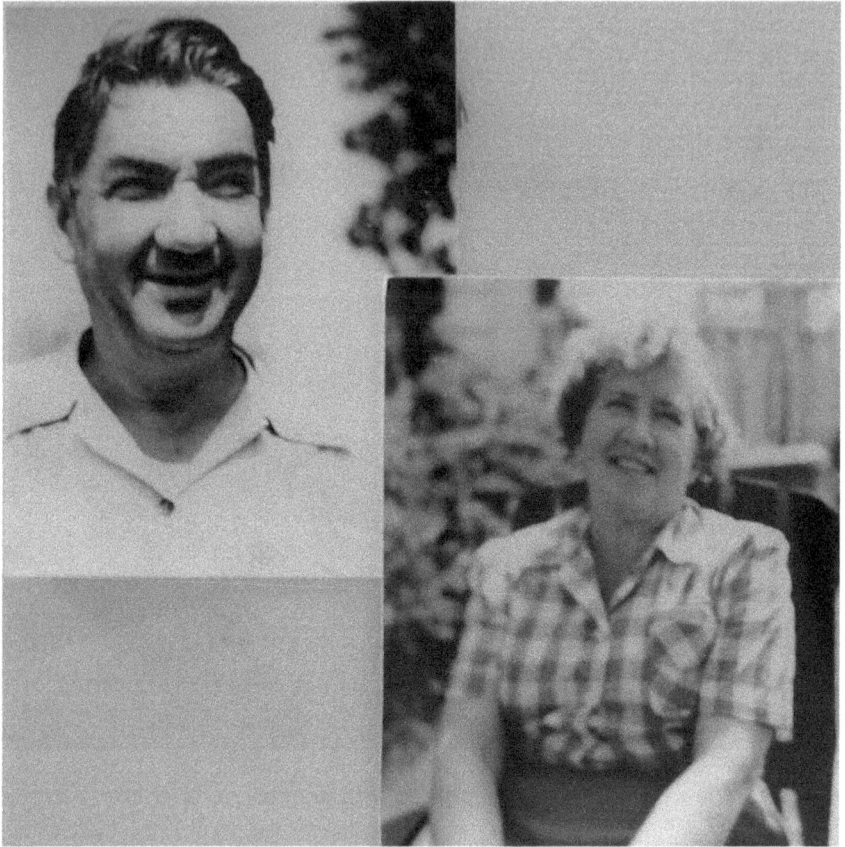

Figure 3.4 Clara Thompson and Henry Major. Reprinted with permission, © William Alanson White Institute.

While Provincetown was a mecca for gay and other unconventional people, the relationship between the Provincetown residents and the summer gay community was not always harmonious. Karen Christel Krahulik (2007) provides a detailed history that follows the town's development, from 1859 to its current reputation as a gay community. Krahulik notes that while Provincetown was a bohemian's paradise, there were many people who held conventional gender ideas. Marlon Brando was reportedly kicked out of his housing "for bringing home too many young sailors" (Manso, 2002, p. 31). Also of that era was Tennessee Williams who was described as enjoying the extraordinary all-night parties on Captain Jack's

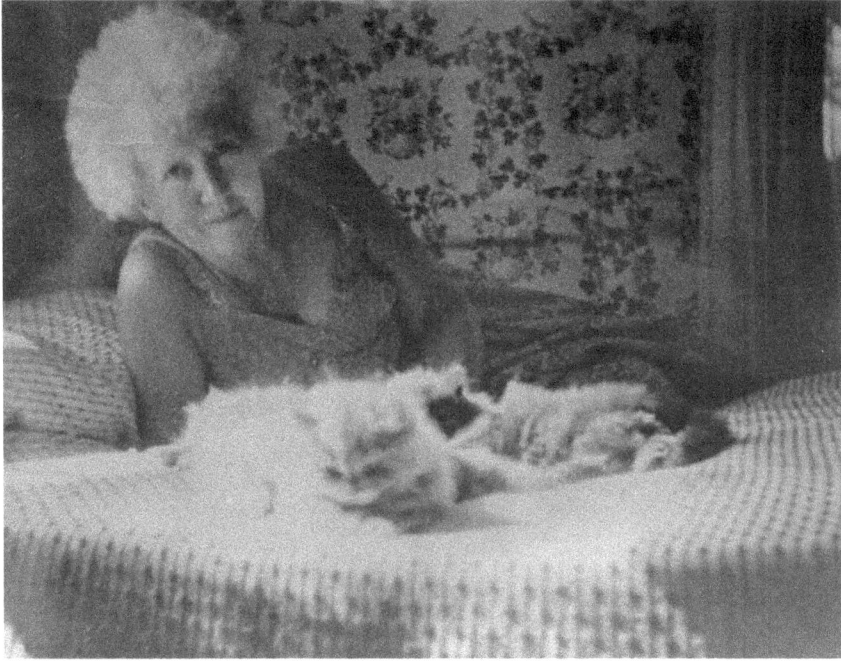

Figure 3.5 Clara Thompson, photo by Gerard Chrzanowski. Reprinted with permission, © William Alanson White Institute.

Wharf. A mixture of acceptance and rejection, conventional and unconventional attitudes, was—and in many ways still is—a part of the fabric of Provincetown.

Letters From Provincetown: Ralph Crowley and Clara Thompson

Ralph Crowley was a student of Harry Stack Sullivan's and close friend of Clara Thompson. Intellectually they each shared the belief "that the human emotional reactions of analysts to their patients not only cannot be avoided, but can be used to facilitate analytic understanding and progress" (Crowley, 1985, p. 336).

Crowley and Thompson were avid letter writers. The trove of handwritten letters between them is held in the Ralph Crowley Papers (Box 3, fol. Series 2) and reprinted with original spelling and punctuations.[3]

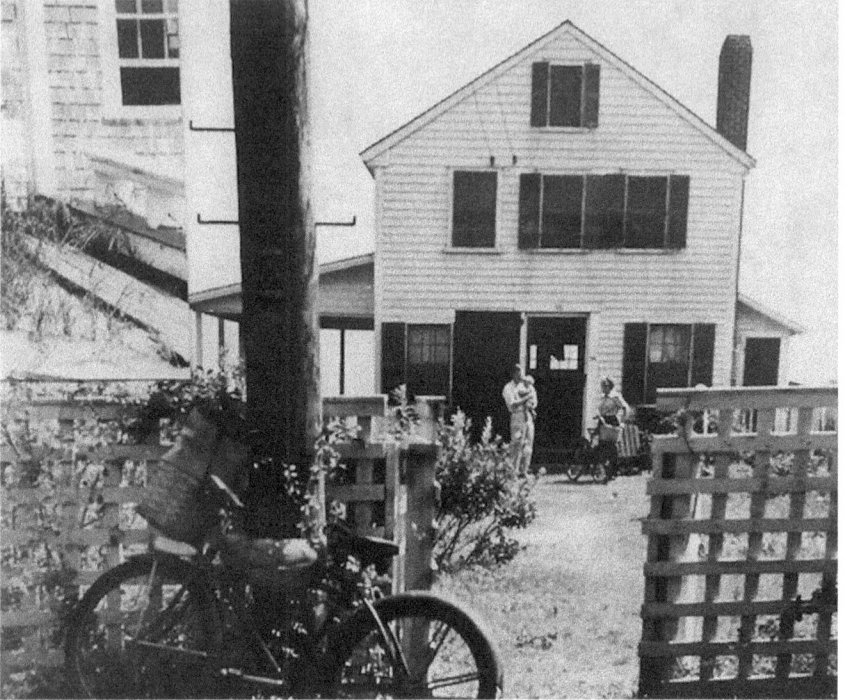

Figure 3.6 Clara Thompson's house in Provincetown. Reprinted with permission, © William Alanson White Institute.

Many of the letters from Provincetown have her Provincetown address (599 Commercial Street, Provincetown, MA) printed on the letterhead. Others, the early ones, use the 151 East 83rd Street, New York address as letterhead. The formality of the stationery is the only formal element of the correspondence. The letters are chatty and conversational, bringing news of the Cape, gossip, health updates, as well as a discussion of institutional issues at first concerning the Washington Society, then the WAW Institute. One gets the feeling while reading these letters that Thompson was involved with coordinating many different groups or people. The expression, "herding cats" comes to mind. I refer the reader to the historian Makari (2008) for more information about the conflicting personalities, ideas, and points of view that appeared during these years.

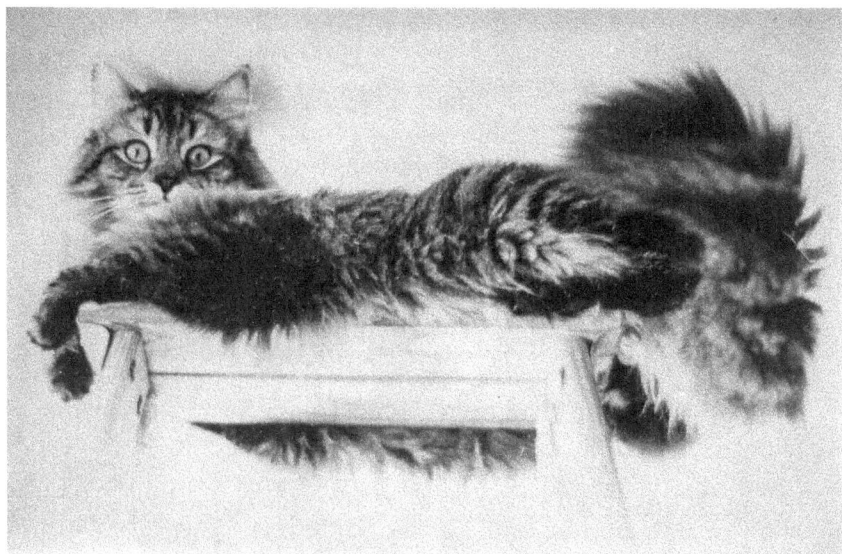

Figure 3.7 Clara Thompson's cat, Mochka. Reprinted with permission, © William Alanson White Institute.

The Letters

August 30, 1945[4]

Dear Ralph

I'm very glad to hear of the rabbit's good sense & look forward to Judith. The food was certainly a blessing. We lived on it for a week believe it or not.

I think I must have given you the impression that the Washington School was planning to start training lay analysts in a kind of irresponsible way. As far as I know the matter has not gone very far yet. There is some agitation in the army for some more adequate training of lay therapists. This is the starting point. We have been thinking that some standardization of what might be considered adequate training for a non-medical therapist might be a way of making some sense out of the present completely unfavorable set up. We would certainly not start it in a big way & there would be very definite standards for pre analytic training. To answer your first objection, we would certainly

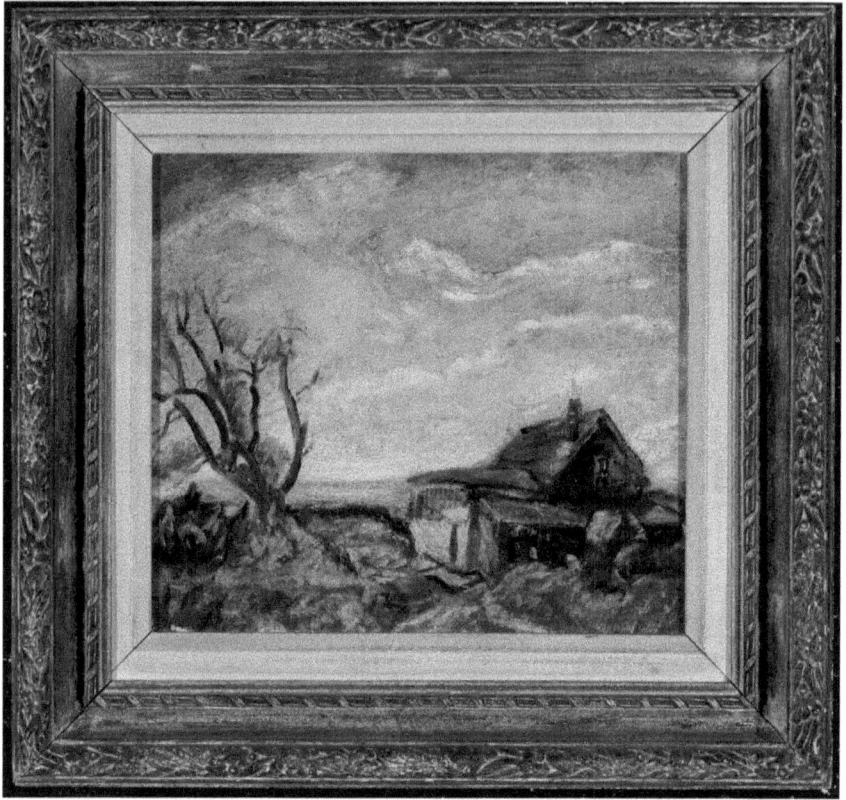

Figure 3.8 Painting by Henry Major; Major, Henry, untitled (a Provincetown scene), n.d., oil on canvas, 14 × 16 in., Gift of Helen K. Snider, 1994. Reprinted with permission of the Provincetown Art Association Museum.

insist on working out some way whereby they could get psychiatric experience in hospitals. It is not impossible that such an arrangement with some hospitals could be worked out we have that in mind. As to the terminology doctor patient etc. well we would probably give it another name. Psychoanalysis it seems to me is becoming thought of less and less as therapy since so many patients today are not really sick in any usual sense.

The second point—what effect it will have on the training of medical men I am sure David Rioch will give plenty of thought to for he more than any of the rest of us is interested in establishing the school

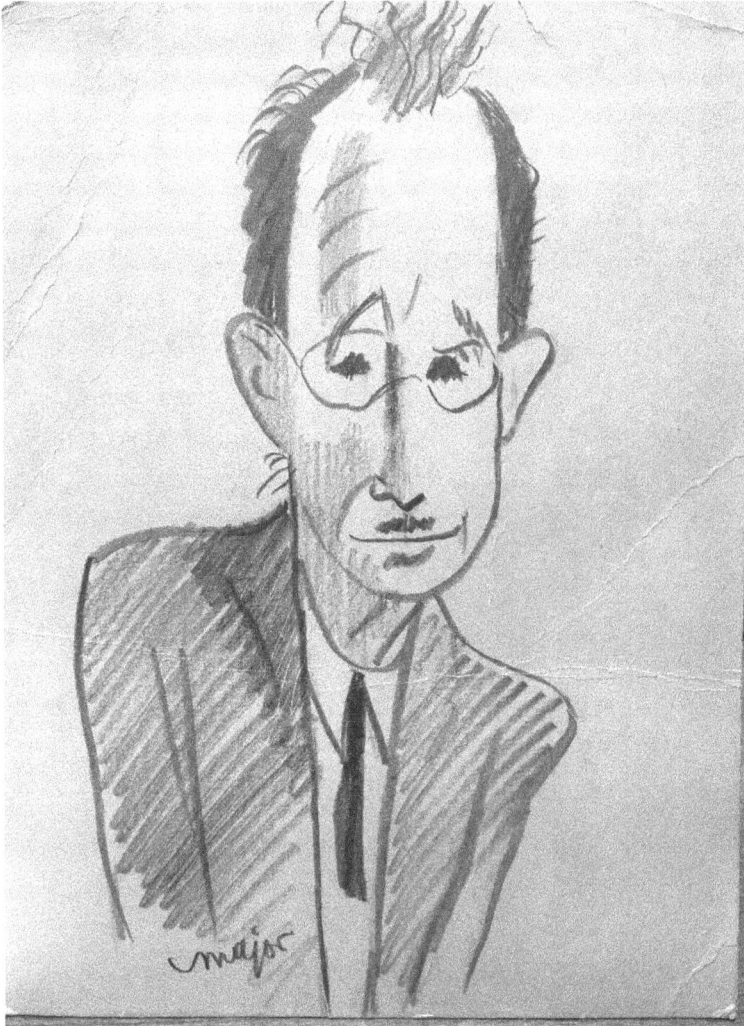

Figure 3.9 Drawing of Harry Stack Sullivan by Henry Major. Reprinted with permission, © William Alanson White Institute.

with good academic standing. Whether other psychoanalytic institutes
recognize our work I think is of less importance since I think we would
consider some of their standards questionable.

I think you are knocking down a straw man in your third point. To
date the school has not taken on any non-medical person to train as a
therapist. The problem of course always is what is a non-therapeutic

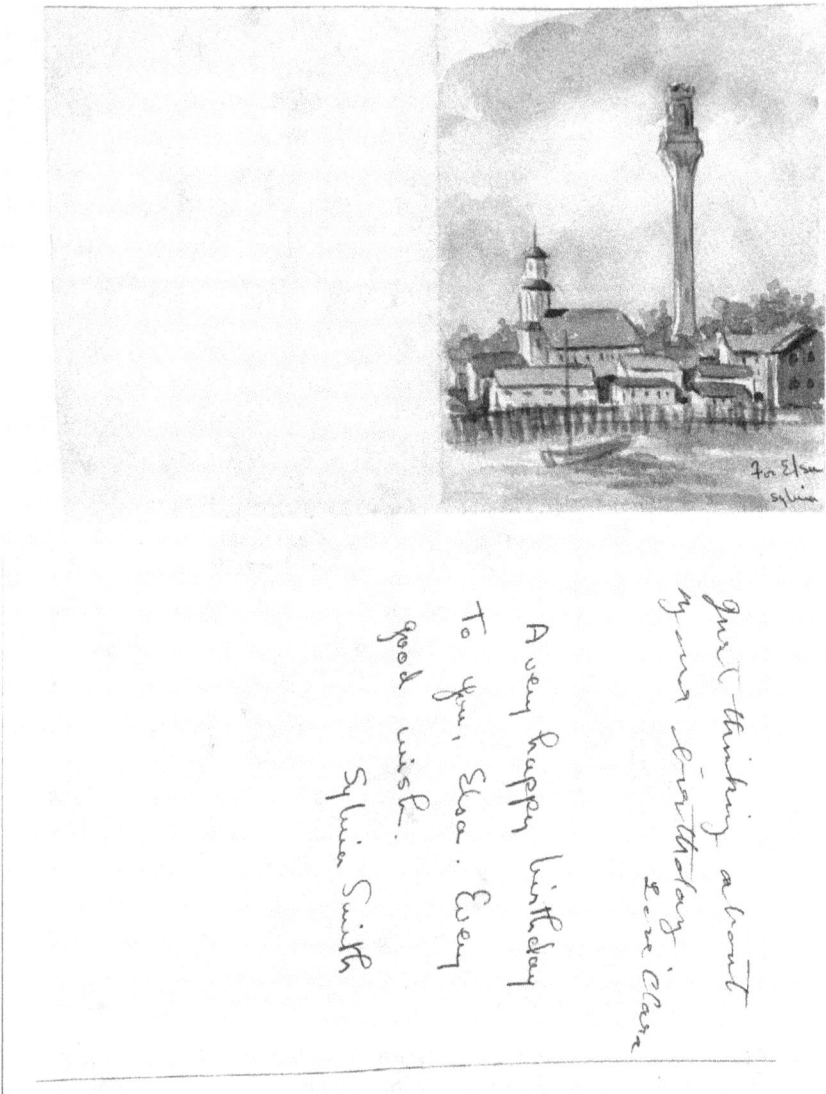

Figure 3.9.i Hand-painted note card by Clara Thompson depicting a view of Provincetown. Reprinted with permission, © William Alanson White Institute.

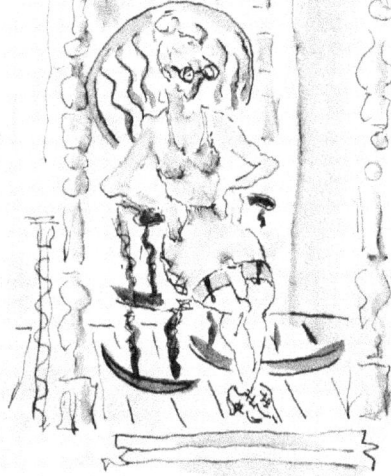

Figure 3.9.ii Hand-painted note card by Clara Thompson: The Girdle Brigade. Reprinted with permission, © William Alanson White Institute.

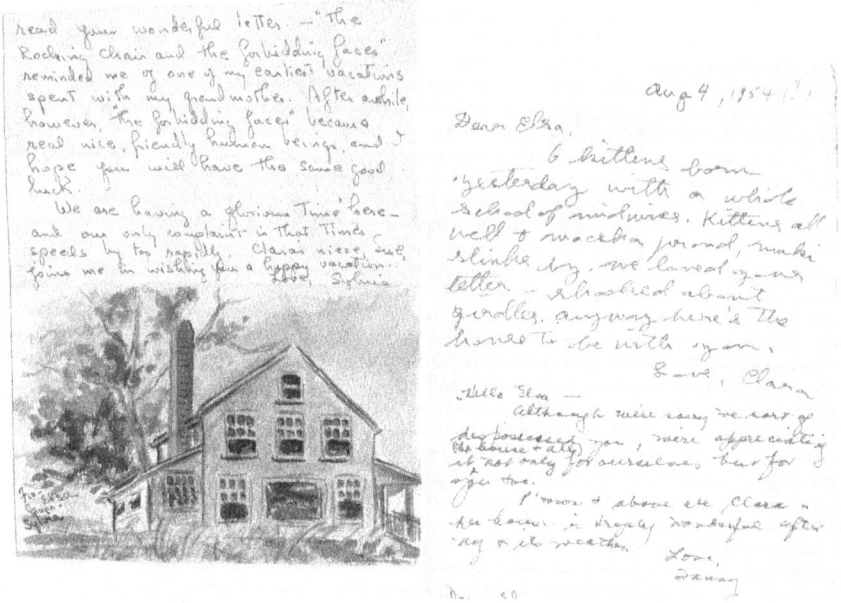

Figure 3.9.iii Hand-painted note card by Clara Thompson depicting Clara's house. Reprinted with permission, © William Alanson White Institute.

relationship since I think we all agree that any analysis undertaken sincerely effects (sic) the character structure favorably. I think Mildred Burye?? is an excellent example of how a clear policy of being in a position to indorse [sic] some people's work & not others would be a great help. She came to me for a therapeutic analysis not for training. Any patient can use her therapist for her own purposes if she is unprincipled enough. Since there is as yet no law against a non-medical person doing what amounts to therapy on his own I don't think we can [missing line] refused to let Mildred take our advanced seminars & we have told her we consider her personality difficulties such that we would not be willing to indorse her even if we did train lay people. Of course, that is a weaker position than if we could say we do train a few selected non-medical people but you do not pass the requirements.

I guess the only point on which you & I would really disagree is this. Why should we shrink from taking responsibility for training certain carefully selected people whose capacities we respect. It seems to me it is just as alarming to take responsibility for training a medical man except that we ourselves feel a little more protected having an established authority to learn on. The fact that a thing has established recognition doesn't necessarily mean it is good & I still would prefer to send a patient to a person I trust than to one with all the credentials in the world whom I don't trust. Are we so far apart. Best Wishes, Clara

The dispute over the training of non-medical therapists is an important issue in the history of psychoanalysis in the United States. It reached a climax at the Washington Society, the Association for the Advancement of Psychoanalysis, and the William Alanson White Institute. Characteristic of Thompson, she shared her opinions in a way that did not intimidate or judge. She was persuasive and collegial.

August 29, 1948
Dear Ralph,

I sure have been slow in answering your letter. It has been a strange summer playing the game with Henry & it has worked pretty well. He is stronger than when he came in June & has had some quite happy days. I don't know whether you read newspapers—on your vacation— if so you may have seen that two days ago his wife was instantly killed in an auto accident. So suddenly after all these years we are free.

To answer your two questions first Erich, Freda & recently Janet have been doing some controls at 15 or more so I see no reason why you should not use your own judgement about it. It does not have to be official. You can say all your student time is taken. I have also resorted to having two in one hour & getting $15 that way.

Secondly about group therapy in the low-cost service. I think your arguments for it are good. I talked to Janet who was here & she raised the question that more of us older people are in a position to supervise it & she would not like to see us do something in a half-baked way with the official backing of the school. So I think we'd better have a faculty meeting about it. She felt it surely should not be in place of a low-cost patient. I don't suppose you have heard from Erich.

I think the report was fine I shall be staying on here probably until October but I shall have a conference with Janet & Ed this week &

I guess the bunch of you can somehow manage for a while. Greetings to peg. Clara

The double life that Major and Thompson were living finally came to a close with the death of Major's wife. Unfortunately, Henry Major was gravely ill, so the time the couple had together free from his marriage was short lived. Weeks later:

September 8, 1948
Dear Ralph
    I thought the enclosed letter was something you might attend to. I think the feeling is we are rather pleased to have Yale interested & so we would like to keep in touch with them. I wrote him to get in touch with you, said I doubted whether we could take anymore persons inventories this fall but we would be glad to talk over with him how he felt we could be useful to him.
    Hope you had a good vacation. Henry continues pretty cheerful & does a little painting nearly every day. He has a pretty hard time breathing now but doesn't notice it much with the drugs he has. Perhaps you read that his wife was killed in an auto accident 10 days ago. It makes the return to N.Y. much simpler. We hope to stay here until Oct.
    Love to Peg & yourself. Clara

In these letters, we hear Thompson discuss the death of Henry Major's wife, Elizabeth Alexander: "They were at last free," and "it made life simpler." She preferred simple, direct language. She once called herself the "Silent Swede," referring to some distant Scandinavian background (Moulton, 1975).

August 12, 1950
Dear Ralph
    The institute seems indeed to be doing well & Virginia when I saw her did not seem too bitter. She seems to comfort herself with the feeling I also am somewhat discarded. I haven't disabused her although I assure you I don't feel that way.
    Edith Wergert is here & will be until the 19th but I've decided not to talk business with her unless she begins it. I think if we are to say

anything about the Washington Society's attitude we should do it as a group & not just one individual here & there shooting off.

By the way, I haven't heard anything about the two problems I left you. Did John Powell answer my letter & did Bibring have any further ideas. I was talking with Finnesinger? last night. He is here. He is now in Baltimore at the In. of Md. He seemed sympathetic with us. At least he expressed himself as puzzled by the attitude of the Baltimore society & did not seem to like the APA's tyranny. I gather he may be starting a training center so he'll have his troubles too. But maybe I'm wrong. It was at a party & everybody was talking across everybody else.

I'm glad Peg is coming along ok. Does she plan to start with me in Oct. still. Eva Maskin seems to be having a great time enjoying her pregnancy. Meyer says he's racing to see if he can have his baby first. He seems to be making good strides on his book. I haven't been working very hard on any new one. I decided I might as well relax & enjoy my present success a little.

Send me the news if you have any.

Affectionately, Clara

August 19, 1950

Dear Ralph

Today I write you about John Powell. Apparently Virginia characteristically considered it too unimportant to show me. I believe also he & Powdermaker did workout some dates. There is I think some correspondence on it but if you can't find it he would certainly know.

What did Hadley write? That seems to be another letter I didn't see?

Do you please get rid of the weights on your mind. I'm impressed with the problems the administrative com. got settled. I imagine you don't really need any opinion but I'm interested to know what is going on.

About Dr. Boardman I do not think I could work with her although I respect her sincerity, & I have tentatively promised R. Trigue if I can find the time. It is sure that I would be much more willing to try to find the time for him then Boardman. So I'm afraid I can't help you on that problem & so according to our custom I guess you'd better keep your secrets about her.

Affectionately, Clara

August 24, 1950

Dear Ralph

I guess John Powell is OK not being a scientist he apparently is susceptible to the frequent misconception that the fact something produces a cure means it is valid. I shall write him in that line & tell him it is ok to go ahead with us.

I'm enclosing a letter from some one Pat recommends. He sounds like a worthwhile problem. Possibly some student would be interested even if we can take him on now.

I showed your letter to Edith. She said she thought the committee had decided not to send out your reprint with the brochure & that accordingly the envelopes were being made to fit the brochure. So I suppose we should abide by the committee.

The typewriter is ok.

I'm surprised about Stevens although I have always had some sort of uneasiness about him—couldn't put my finger on it—too smooth. Anyway I think we should reconsider his case. In the meantime let him take basic courses.

Very sorry about Peg. Love Clara

In the aftermath of the Second World War, many psychoanalysts had immigrated the United States. The following letter mentions the status of foreign students with immigration visas.

August 30, 1950

Dear Ralph

I am returning Powell's letter for the files & Hadley's letter. I had not seen it it must have arrived the day after I left. It might be worth while to check with Billy Silverberg because he must be in the same boat & it would be good to know what he plans to do.

I think both Ferguson & Mendelsohn do not come under the foreign student situation since both of them are here on immigration visas since it was the only way they could come at the time.

Give my love to Peggy.

Clara

August 15, 1954

Dear Ralph

I suppose by now you have heard that Ernest Hadley died I think probably on Aug. 9. I don't know what happened. I received a telegram but that was after I heard of it from the Times. So I haven't done anything about the letter we all received. We'll doubtless hear more in time. I thought maybe the Inst. should send his wife condolences but it seems so hypocritical I haven't been able to make myself tell Lloyd. If you think we ought to do something in terms of public relations will you drop a line to Lloyd or send a telegram yourself as acting director.

About your resignation. I don't want to press you because I think your devotion to the institute is amply demonstratable & that you do carry a terrific load. I suppose the election of a substitute is up to the Fellows. Janet certainly has a lot to offer but do you have any reason to think she would accept. Another possibility is Meyer who since his marriage is once more friendly with Ed. Janet & Ed don't hit it off well. I sort of shudder at having such tension in such a small group. Of course I'd be very happy if you reconsidered. Anyway have a good vacation. I've had a lot of company but have also managed to get the anthology done.

Love to you & Peggy

Clara

July 24, 1956

Dear Ralph

Many thanks for your care of my garden.

Your idea of planning committee is fine & I agree to the choice. In the absence of Ed don't you think the two of us as exec. com. could appoint it proterm & confirm later. Also I agree with your project. Could you have everything ready & then we could have a meeting of the trustees Sept. 18. But if that's too late I'll call it whenever you wish and Mac Loyd can preside. My vote is for the 12,500. I understand Fromm plans to be in N.Y. the last 2 weeks in Sept. He would help make a quorum if he could be persuaded to go to trustees meeting. However probably a quorum isn't too important because decisions could be made & confirmed later. I guess you need a vacation alright. Damn B!

Affectionately Clara

August 19, 1956

Dear Ralph

You didn't say whether Sept. 18 is too late for trustees meeting—so I'm telling Lloyd to send out notices. She says she will be in town about a week around the 1st of Sept. Summer has gone very peacefully for me I have been more lazy than usual enjoying reading & my kittens which are a riot at present.

About Joe he puts up a very good surface socially but when alone he often has that smart crampy look. I tease him about it his profound thoughts & he snaps right out of it. He seems to be studying for his boards pretty adequately. I keep the relationship pretty impersonal & asked nothing of him except to carry his end of the household chores which he seems glad to do. There is no danger of his getting too much attention because Fanny and Sylvia are here & we usually do things as a foursome. So maybe seeing you & being impersonally mothered by me does help him float. As to what goes on inside I haven't the foggiest notion & whenever he tries to talk about it he seems utterly unable to say anything clearly.

About Mrs Russell—I think she is distinctly better—less tense. She dropped in one evening & it was quite pleasant except one of the guests said after she had left "I got completely exhausted responding to her forced smile" and that is still very much in evidence.

And so another summer is ending & I'll be seeing you before long.

My greetings to Peg. Clara

August 11, 1957

Dear Ralph

Your trip sounded wonderful but I suppose by now you are deep in Institute affairs. My summer is quiet & peaceful—sunny days, lovely swimming—a garden in which grow the biggest zucchinis you ever saw—to say nothing of other things. The people in Mexico don't seem to have been especially impressed by their earth quake. At least to date I have tried in vain to get some description of it out of someone. Maybe Zen Buddhism affects you that way—who knows. The usual crowd seems to be milling around here—Zapf. Chrzanowski, Goldensohn, Alt. Mendelsohn, English etc. Anyway if there's anything I can do for 12 E let me know. Affectionately, Clara

July 7, 1958

Dear Ralph

Something certainly seems to be going on with those dreams. Could you be saying in killing your mother you have to die. Then you prove it isn't so. You may be bloody but unbowed. Why does Edith get you so. She knows a lot about administration. Maybe if you just listened & then thought it over you could use what is useful to you. I know she has taught me a lot. At the same time I have never fallen for a hyper-organized institute. Lloyd & Gene seemed to enjoy it here this past weekend. I was a little worried—it is so unMerrile like—here. Milt seems to be working out ok don't you think? I'm much better. I still itch but the flu-like general feeling of sickness has gone.

Write me when you feel like it.

Affectionately, Clara

My best to Pricilla. Incidental intelligence we have 4 kittens, 2 grays & 2 buffs.

July 31, 1958

Dear Ralph

Well I suppose you'll be back at the old stand either tomorrow or Monday. I'm still sort of an invalid. The shingles left me with a new neuritis which is damned uncomfortable but for the last three days that seems to be greatly improved—so I have hopes. One trouble with this disease is everybody who comes along has a sure cure for it & they're all different. So I spend my time trying to drive off would be helpful friends. I have taken so many drugs that my stomach finally protested. So today I'm saying to hell with them all.

Your discoveries about your relations to Priscilla are very interesting. I wonder how it will come out. My reaction to your dream of the two horses was one was one is Pris & one is Peggy. Why should Pris be 2 horses. Have you thought maybe you don't want either & that there may be a better woman in the sense of more united to you just around the corner. I just don't see why it should be either or. Why not be a Bachelor for a while. Can you get something across to Milt about his belittling our point of view? I didn't think he had it as bad as Earl but maybe he has.

Let's know the news of the town when you have collected it.

Affectionately Clara

By the way has Priscilla decided to go on with analysis with me. She seemed in doubt when I left & I'd like to know definitely over one of these days.

August 16, 1958
Dear Ralph

I enclose your excellent report with only one suggestion on page 3. You seem to be achieving real growth in your personal life. More power to you.

About Nechim's proposal get as much information about it as you can. It will have to be brought to the fellows & approved by the Trustees—so you should have a good plan first.

My shingles hang on. I had three fine days this week & thought it was really over but yesterday (with the humidity I suppose) it came back again—the itching I mean. Well it will surely stop someday I suppose & it isn't as bad as it was. I sure am glad it didn't happen during the work year.

Give my greetings to anyone around. A lot are around here— Wittenburg, Singer, English, Braun, Burchard, Arieti—probably more—can't think of them now.

Affectionately Clara

These letters, written between 1945 and the year of her death, 1958, are intimate and detailed. Read together, they convey a tone of cheerfulness that slowly is replaced by the somberness of illness and death.

Thompson's quiet attunement is revealed in a story told by her former student, the psychoanalyst Edgar Levenson (2017). He recalls tells his summer visit to the Cape and Thompson's expression of empathy.

One summer my wife and I and our two in diapers (13 months apart) children were staying in a rental house in Wellfleet on the Cape. We were at a party at Clara's in Provincetown when she said to me, "What's the matter? You two look exhausted." Actually, we were close to suicide because both babies screamed all night, one setting off the other, in the modernistic beach house we'd rented more for its looks than its practicality . . . the next day a car bumped up the drive at our place in Wellfleet and out came Clara . . . she sat with us for an hour, chatted pleasantly, and then left. Nothing was said about children or our despair—she just kept us company. I was really touched, because it was not easy for her to get around, but also by the way she engaged with us. It was very much her style: this nonverbal empathic recognition and response, without formulation and explanation. Oddly I found it especially comforting.

(p. 30)

Levenson also described spending time with colleagues on the Cape: "Actually Erwin, Ben Wolstein, and I spent a lot of time together, particularly on the Cape, with Ed Tauber present. Ben always managed to somehow leave out that his first analysis was with Ed Tauber. He had a real falling out with Ed years later and he sort of made him persona non grata and claimed his major influence was from Clara Thompson. But we used to spend a lot of time sitting around on the Cape talking about theoretical stuff" (Hirsch & Iannuzzi, 2004, p. 257).

The psychoanalysts Paul and Frances Lippmann recall visits to Provincetown when Ruth Moulton and Louis Gilbert were there. They heard tales of Clara's parties that ran late into the night, where alcohol flowed freely, and of the beach adventures, where sandy bare feet were *de rigueur*. Lippmann also recalls two other WAW analysts who were regulars: Erwin Singer, who owned a gay guest house across the street from a center of town restaurant, Bubalas, and Woody English, who lived in North Truro on Depot Road.

Provincetown Remembers Thompson

Thompson is buried in Provincetown's Protestant cemetery; her striking headstone was sculpted by Philip Malicoat's son Conrad. It is soft and abundant, bold, and soaring, reaching up toward the clouds. Opposite her grave is that of Henry Major. He too has a prominent sculpture that bears an inscription, most likely written by Thompson: "He has taught men a respect for life." Each year on the anniversary of Henry Major's death, Thompson met with a group of his friends at his grave site.

A respect for life and a zest for living unfettered by conformity is Thompson's Provincetown legacy. She chose the right place when she made her home on Commercial Street over two decades before her death. Her house is featured in the iconic book *Building Provincetown: A Guide to Its Social and Cultural History Told Through Its Architecture* (Dunlap, 2015). Provincetown has not forgotten Clara Mabel Thompson.

Notes

1 John (Ike) Taylor Williams, a prominent Boston literary agent.
2 Fanny's surname was not included.
3 While many people are referenced in these letters, I've made only a modest attempt to discover what role they may have played at the William Alanson White Institute.
4 Thompson, C. (1945–1958). Letters to Ralph Crowley. The Oskar Diethelm Library, DeWitt Wallace Institute Psychiatry: History, Policy, & the Arts, Weill Cornell Medical College, The Ralph Crowley Papers, Box 3, Folder 1, New York, NY.

References

Ben-Zvi, L. (2005). *Susan Glaspell: Her life and times*. Oxford and New York: Oxford University Press.

Crowley, R. (1985). Selected writings. *Contemporary Psychoanalysis*, 21, 336–345.

Cunningham, M. (2002). *Land's end: A walk in Provincetown*. New York: Crown.

D'Ercole, A. (2017). On finding Clara Thompson. *Contemporary Psychoanalysis*, *53*(1), 63–68.

Dunlap, D. W. (2015). *Building Provincetown: A guide to its social and cultural history told through its architecture*. Provincetown, MA: Provincetown Historical Commission.

Green, M. R. (1964). Her life. In M. R. Green (Ed.), *Interpersonal psychoanalysis: The selected papers of Clara M. Thompson*. New York: Basic Books.

Hirsch, I., & Iannuzzi, V. (2004). Interview with Edgar A. Levenson. *Contemporary Psychoanalysis*, *41*(4), 593–644.

Krahulik, K. C. (2007). *Provincetown: From pilgrim landing to gay resort*. New York: New York University Press.

Levenson, E. A. (2017). *Interpersonal psychoanalysis and the enigma of consciousness*. London: Routledge.

Major, H. (1948, September 23). Henry Major obituary. *Provincetown Advocate*.

Makari, G. (2008). *Revolution in mind: The creation of psychoanalysis*. Harper Collins, New York.

Manso, P. (2002). *Ptown: Art, sex, and money on the outer cape*. New York: Simon & Schuster.

Moulton, R. (1969). My memories of being supervised. *Contemporary Psychoanalysis*, *5*(2), 151–157.

Moulton, R. (1975). Early papers on women: Horney to Thompson. *American Journal of Psychoanalysis*, *35*(3), 207–223.

Porter, A. (2009). *Kasztner's train: The true story of an unknown hero of the holocaust*. New York: Walker & Company.

The Provincetown Advocate. (1948, September 23). Obituary: "Henry Major dies was noted artist." https://encore.clamsnet.org/iii/encore/search/C__SThe%20 advocate__Orightresult__U?lang=eng&suite=def

Provincetown Art Association. (1938). *Provincetown art association: 1938 Annual exhibition.* Provincetown History Preservation Project. Retrieved from http://provincetownhistoryproject.com/PDF/059_276_578b-018-province-town-art-association-exhibition-1938.pdf

Provincetown Art Association. (1939). Provincetown art association: Second 1939 annual exhibition. Twenty-Fifth Season. Provincetown History Preservation Project.

Scutts, J. (2019, November 25). Feminize your canon: Mary Heaton Vorse. *The Paris Review.* Strick&Williams, Tierra Innovation, and the staff of *The Paris Review.* ©2016 *The Paris Review.*

Sprague, C. (2001, August 2). Explorer of inner space: Groundbreaking psychoanalyst made her home here. *Provincetown Banner*, pp. 37–41.

Thompson, C. (1945–1958). Letters to Ralph Crowley. The Oskar Diethelm Library, DeWitt Wallace institute psychiatry: History. Policy, & the Arts, Weill Cornell Medical College, The Ralph Crowley Papers, Box 4, folder 10, New York, NY.

Thompson, C. (1945) Transference as a therapeutic instrument. *Psychiatry*, 8, 273–278.

Thompson, C. (1947). Changing concepts of homosexuality in psychoanalysis. *Psychiatry*, X, 183–189.

Thompson, C. (1950). *Psychoanalysis evolution and development.* New York: Basic Books.

Thompson, C. (1964) Memorial Service February 11, 1949 in M. R. Green, Her life. Green, M. R. Interpersonal Psychoanalysis Selected Papers of Clara M. Thompson. Basic Books, New York.

Taylor Williams, J. (2022). *The Shores of Bohemia—Radicals on the outer cape, 1910–1960* Farrar, Strauss & Giroux, 2022.

Chapter 4

Creating a Tradition
Bringing the Past to the Future

In 1920, the year Clara Thompson completed medical school, the field of psychoanalysis was about 20 years old. Thompson (1950) reviews the history of the shifts from Freud to the culturalists of her generation in her essay:

> The workers in the earlier years concentrated on finding more effective methods of therapy and on trying to enlarge the therapeutic scope of psychoanalysis. There was a shift in emphasis from concern with recall of the past (the removal of the infantile amnesia) to the understanding of the dynamics of the doctor-patient relationship as observed in treatment. This interest did not disappear after 1934; it became embodied in Sullivan's theory of interpersonal relations. Increased study of comparative culture in the later 1920s eventually contributed significantly to another challenging of Freud's biological theory of neurosis by the so-called cultural school of analysts, whose thinking began to influence psychoanalysis around 1934.
>
> (1950a, p. 5)

Thompson's scholarly contributions began in 1930. She was honing her therapeutic approach over the summer months she was in analysis with Sándor Ferenczi and throughout the rest of the year as she was involved with her American colleagues, including Harry Stack Sullivan in Baltimore. There were weekly meetings of the "Miracle Club," a supervision and social gathering that helped her work with her patients. Then in New York, Thompson, Horney, Sullivan, and Fromm met regularly, each helping to establish an American psychoanalytic tradition. She explained that American psychiatrists understood the importance of the environment as a contributing factor in illness; they were also less literal than their European

DOI: 10.4324/9781003284840-5

counterparts in the way they applied Freud's theories. Both Ferenczi and Sullivan had maintained that an active technique was helpful in treating character problems, as was an awareness of the interaction between the analyst and patient. Thompson (1950a) recalls,

> A few analysts were showing interest in learning about the relations of man to his society by a collaboration with anthropologists and sociologists in the study of comparative cultures.
>
> (p. 195)

Initially conceptualized by 19th-century anthropologists, "participant observation" as a concept made its way from anthropology into the psychoanalytic canon (D'Ercole, 2017, p. 95). It was a central idea in the original interpersonal tradition underscoring the mutually influencing and influential aspects of any interpersonal encounter. With this interdisciplinary legacy as background, along with her experience with Ferenczi, Thompson, and Sullivan, along with Erich Fromm and Karen Horney, joined forces with social scientists like Edward Sapir and Ruth Benedict. Together they considered how learned defensive patterns in interpersonal relationships and unconscious identifications influenced the complex interactions between the patient and analyst. Thompson (1952) believed the clinical encounter was about the patient and the analyst and the patient together. Maurice Green (1964a) gathered a collection of Thompson's articles and unpublished paper presentations in *Interpersonal Psychoanalysis: The Selected Papers of Clara Mabel Thompson*. Regarding Thompson's contributions to what came to be known as interpersonal psychoanalysis, he wrote,

> her emphasis, in theory as well as practice, was always concentrating on and analyzing what went on between persons to facilitate the growth of a human relationship—what I would call interpersonal psychoanalysis.
>
> (p. vii)

Thompson, however, used the terms "interpersonal relations" (1978, p. 492; 1988, p. 194; 2017, p. 8), "interpersonal theory" (2017, p. 11), "interpersonal process" (1978, p. 496), and "interpersonal forces" (1978, p. 50) in her writings. Green's (1964b) essential albeit brief biographical essay at the end of the collection provides information about Thompson's life that would otherwise not exist. I have drawn liberally from it throughout this biography.

Missing in Action: The Limits of Psychoanalytic Electronic Publishing (PEP)

Outside of Green's (1964a) edited volume, Thompson's articles can be difficult to locate. Using the term "Thompson, Clara" in a PEP web search (as of 10/06/2019) produced 71 original citations. Within that search, most are in the form of book reviews or summaries of papers. Some of those reviews contain a few pithy lines, while others are longer, offering opinions about the work.

These reviews, while not the whole of her *oeuvre*, are significant. They provide her perspective on current topics in the field. A sense of Thompson's breadth of psychoanalytic knowledge emerges.[1]

In her review of Schilder's (1938) essay *"Psychoanalysis and Conditioned Reflexes,"* Thompson (1938a) suggests:

> The term reflex is a bad name, for the facts concern a different level of the animals' psyche. It is important that physiological understanding and psychological should agree. Pavlov's data is valuable but his physiology is pseudo-physiology. To accept it one must give up the idea of the personality as a whole and configurations.
>
> Analysts are mistaken in feeling the need of corroboration of their work from Pavlov's field. His animal experimentation, on the other hand, does not need corroboration from the psychological side, but, in invading the field of higher nervous activity, his work cannot be valid when it contradicts acknowledged results in that field.
>
> (p. 101)

In Thompson's (1946) review of *Conceptual Thinking in Schizophrenia* by Hanfmann and Kasanin (1942), she offers positive thoughts but ends with a strong critique.

> The book is well-organized and well written. The research seems carefully planned and executed and the conclusions are convincing. The only criticism is the one which can be made concerning the application

of laboratory methods to human behavior generally. For example, on what basis was it determined that a subject was normal. Also is it not possible that the same schizophrenics at another stage of their illness would have shown different results!"

(1946, p. 384)

Thompson (1940a) does not shy away from offering criticism. Her review of Kamiat's (1939) *Social Forces in Personality Stunting* provides an opportunity to see how she argues her objections to the work. She maintains,

> The title of this book is misleading. Although the aim as stated is to show that the cause of personal immaturity is the stunting effect of the "exploitative, autocratic and competitive" spirit of society, actually the main thesis of the book is the exact opposite.
>
> (p. 572)

Unfortunately, only four of her authored articles listed in the PEP web search were published during her lifetime: "Analytic Observations During the Course of a Manic-Depressive Psychosis" (1930); " 'Dutiful Child' Resistance" (1931); "Identification with the Enemy and Loss of the Sense of Self" (1940b); and "The Therapeutic Technique of Sándor Ferenczi: A Comment" (1943). One might stop there, thinking that was the sum total of her contributions to the literature. Adding "The Dynamics of Hostility" (1959a); the Spanish version of "Un Estudio del Clima Emocional de los Institutos Psicoanalíticos (1959b); "Sullivan and Psychoanalysis" (1978); "Sullivan and Fromm" (1979); "Sándor Ferenczi" (1988); and "The History of the William Alanson White Institute" (2017), all published after her death, offer only a partial view of her published contributions to the field.

A PEP web search does not include essays published in the journal *Psychiatry* and other journals and books where she published. That includes her review of Ferenczi's *Thalassa, A Theory of Genitality* (1939) and significantly, her important papers "The Role of Women in This Culture" (1941); "Cultural Pressures in the Psychology of Women" (1942); " 'Penis Envy' in Women" (1943a); "Transference as a Therapeutic Instrument" (1945); "Changing Concepts of Homosexuality in Psychoanalysis" (1947); "Cultural Conflicts of Women in Our Society" (1949); "Some Effects of the Derogatory Attitude Toward Female Sexuality" (1950b); "A Study of the Emotional Climate of Psychoanalytic Institutes" (1958b); and "An Introduction to Minor Maladjustments" (1959c). Still, this is only a partial listing of her publications (see bibliography from Green, 1964a).

On Reading Thompson

It is best to begin reading Thompson in her book, *Psychoanalysis: Evolution and Development* (1950a). It is a *tour de force* that grew from student requests for copies of her lectures presented at various schools and institutes, including Johns Hopkins Medical School, New York Medical College, New York Psychoanalytic Institute, New School for Social Research, Washington School of Psychiatry, and William Alanson White Institute of Psychiatry.

My copy features a photo of Thompson on the back jacket. Dust jackets are now largely passe, for academic books however in their day, they did more than protect books from dust. Thompson's was written by the American writer and poet, Millen Brand. Brand was best known for his widely popular screenplay, *Snake Pit*.[2] An interesting side note, Chrzanowski, Thompson's close colleague, was used as the therapist's model in the film *Snake Pit*. Inside the front flap, he describes the book:

> *Psychoanalysis: Evolution and Development* is the first simple and comprehensive survey of all of Freud's work and theory, along with a tolerant and balanced account of the more important divergent schools of psychoanalytic thought. The general reader who wants to know, what is largely the unknown Freud, the Freud of the later stage when he was veering away from sex and examining the forces of death and aggression brought home to him by the First World War, will find the full story here. Dr. Thompson recalls to us that the contemporary cultural approach to psychoanalysis had its deep roots in Freud's own thinking, and that there is not quite the difference among the analytic schools that the extreme deviants want us to believe. . . . In terms of its inclusive review of "theory and therapy" it is hard to overemphasize the importance of this clear, tolerant, unifying book, the first handbook of psychoanalysis. . . . Through this book we recognize its growing importance as a general force behind the good life, and as an instrument through which, sanely and generously, we may find ourselves in others, and others in ourselves.

The book's opening sentences reveal Thompson's quiet rebellious nature and are remarkable for their insightfulness: "Psychoanalysis did not spring full grown from the brow of Freud. It has a history" (p. 3). With that one sentence, she rejects the 19th-century "Great Man Theory" by Thomas Carlyle (1841), which argued that history could be explained by the impact of great men, heroes, or highly influential individuals. Instead, with cheekiness she dismisses this now largely discredited theory. Instead, she argues:

> psychoanalysis emerged under the stress of practical exigencies, it shows gaps, regressions and bypaths, as well as progressions. Hence, a historical survey of analysis is necessary for a thorough understanding. . . . Psychoanalysis is, first of all, a method and technique of therapy for mental and emotional disorder, around which there has evolved a definite body of theory.
>
> (1950a, p. 3)

Like her essays, the book sometimes reads as a conversation one can imagine having with her about Freud and his descendants:

> Whatever one may think of Freud's theoretical orientation, he made the enormously significant discovery that childhood experiences are of the greatest importance for subsequent personality development; and that the effects of such experiences continue to operate outside conscious awareness. It happened that his first discoveries were made in connection with hysteria where strong early sexual interests accompanied by strong prohibitions against them are frequently discovered as originating factors. Hysteria is seen much less frequently today; it seems possible that cultural changes account to some extent for its disappearance, and that it is more prominent whenever the sexual life is hedged in as it was in the Victorian era. At any rate, the frequency of hysteria in his patients during the years when Freud was first formulating his theories may well have been the decisive influence in bringing to his attention the significance of repressed sexuality in neurosis.
>
> Freud's turning away from environmental factors, as a major concern, to organic constitution was, however, most unfortunate. For this reason, he came to minimize what actually happens between people, failed to take into consideration what more recent observations

suggests, that it is the dynamic interaction between people which provides the locus of functional mental illness.

(pp. 26–27)

In a moment of modest self-reflection, Thompson shared with her friend, the psychoanalyst Zeborah Schachtel, that "she did not think of herself as an intellectual, nor a therapist." Instead, she mused, "she just said what she thought" (personal communication, May 2016). This characterization of herself that may lead some mistakenly to undervalue her contributions.

Published Essays

When read together, the four essays published between 1930 and 1940, "Analytic Observations During the Course of a Manic-Depressive Psychosis" (1930); "'Dutiful Child' Resistance" (1931); "Development of Awareness of Transference in a Markedly Detached Personality" (1938b); and "Identification with the Enemy and Loss of Sense of Self" (1940b), provide evidence that Thompson was developing a vital object-relational concept in her work with patients. Together they demonstrate her understanding of the importance of the repetition of childhood relational patterns and how identification with hostile parents can suffocate individual growth. She is mindful of how these patterns resurface in analytic treatment and uses them to illustrate her conception of transference and countertransference.

Each essay stressed an important pattern in early childhood relationships. Those relationships, she argues, can establish, and perpetuate destructive and repetitive unconscious processes in later life. In two of those essays, she draws from the case of Marian, a patient in her early 20s.

Patient Marian

Thompson illustrates how "identification with the hated parent" results in a form of contempt that becomes aggression turned against the self. Despite Thompson's intensive efforts Marian sadly committed suicide. Thompson mentions her struggle in working with the patient in a 1932 letter to Izette de Forest:

I've had one tragedy this year. My psychotic patient is having another psychosis. I wish I knew why. Following Ferenczi's method I have tried to find a fault in me and doubtless it is but Ferenczi thinks now that perhaps psychotics need more security than any human being can give them. I know that my being in analysis may have been very hard for her but she was like a baby in reacting to the deep undercurrents in me and I know that she became ill in a very difficult time in my analysis. That is the nearest I can come to my fault.

(Brennan, 2009, p. 447)

The richly detailed clinical case of Marian, presented in "Analytic Observations During the Course of a Manic-Depressive Psychosis" (1930), was Thompson's second paper drawing on that case material. Green (1964a) tells the reader that the first paper, "Identification with the Enemy and Loss of Sense of Self" (1940b), was published in *Psychoanalytic Quarterly* a decade after it was written. It is unclear why it took so long to publish, except for the note that "The final course of this case shows that the original diagnosis was a mistake. This is clearly a case of schizophrenia" (p. 40).

We don't know why she thought it necessary to change the patient's diagnosis to something more serious. Was blaming her patient for a more serious illness an attempt to distance herself from her haunting guilt? Was the change in diagnosis muddled with her unresolved countertransference toward her patient's homosexuality?

In the paper, the reader learns about Marian's sexuality and her cycles of manic-depressive episodes. Marian saw Thompson three times a week for a period, six times a week at another point, and sometimes the patient reportedly did not come for months. Thompson gives a detailed description of the patient's developmental history, making clear that the patient's father was obsessional and "pedantic," pressuring his children to make a good impression. Marian recalled a childhood where she agonized over "doing the wrong thing." Marian's mother was much more disturbed. Her symptoms became evident following Marian's birth and were exacerbated after the birth of a second child, a sister named Sylvia. Marian's mother then ceased to participate in "normal" life. She became "preoccupied with sex," and thinking that all men aimed to seduce her, accused them directly. She spoke "freely" of these episodes with her daughter and warned her child against becoming a prostitute, saying that she would probably either "be that or go crazy" (pp. 240–241).

The patient's mother was institutionalized and within a few years committed suicide. Shortly afterward, the father left and placed his daughters in schools. Marian was 17 the year her mother killed herself; it was also the year she entered college.

Thompson writes:

> In college she made the acquaintance of a girl [Olga] with whom for the first time in her life she felt at ease. . . . On the night of the mother's death they spent the night together. . . . When Marian learned of her mother's death the next morning she was impressed with the coincidence and felt this girl must take the mother's place . . . the girl belonged to a social group which her family considered inferior to theirs. Thus, a feeling of superiority made Marian feel at ease, but at the same time the situation minimized Olga's adoration of her, and she was in the position again of having a mother of whom she was ashamed. As the friendship gradually developed, she was happier than at any time in her life. She felt loved and valued, and as yet no consciousness of conflict had entered. Then they began to room together, and the custom of kissing passionately developed. Marian began to wake nauseated in the morning. This seemed to have something to do with dirty stockings associated with Olga's social status and something wrong about their relationship. The sense of critical eyes of the world increased. She felt she could not pass her examinations—she began to worry about the future, and felt she could never earn her living, that she had no brains. She actually became unable to concentrate and talked constantly of suicide . . . she was placed in a hospital and analytic contact began.
>
> (pp. 241–243)

Marian's sexual conflicts were palpable. Her hospitalization brought her into treatment with Thompson. Immediately, Marian's attachment was intense as Thompson explains how the patient's "transference was marked by a fairly sudden transition from depression to elation—(p. 244)

> Everything now had become all right, sexual fantasies were to be indulged in, masturbation was acceptable. The difficulty was that the elation immediately carried her beyond analytic reach. It served as an effective resistance to analysis, blocking it for some months at the same time that it was the incorporation of the analyst—one might say whole and undigested.
>
> (p. 244)

Thinking about the patient's sexuality, Thompson questions why "the homosexual situation on three separate occasions precipitated depression" (p. 245). She wonders if the patient was "testing the analyst out on the subject":

> At last after three months she told of the homosexual episode, which she had consciously withheld; at the time when she told it she felt it was of no importance and had no emotion concerning it. On the night following this she dreamed of the analyst injecting something into her arm, which brought up the possibility of sexual factors in the transference.
>
> She then began to improve a little and started some occupation to fill her time. In her work she was thrown with a group of young people of less education than herself, and they at once looked upon her as somewhat of a leader, so she found herself for the first time in her life in a limelight, and with young men friendly to her. Her dreams at this time were chiefly of homosexual situations in which her sister as well as Olga figured, but her conscious interest was more and more occupied with the young men in her little social group. These two factors were important in producing again a sudden swing to elation six months after the beginning of analysis the second time. That is—the possibility of a new object love in the homosexual realm was threatening to break into her consciousness in relation to the analyst.
>
> At this time the patient reported some heterosexual successes with boys she despised, they offered a means of escape from the transference.
>
> (pp. 245–246)

Thompson concludes:

> There seems little doubt that her heterosexual interest was exaggerated, and in reality, her success in that sphere was not as great as she tried to believe, and would have the analyst believe. It was an attempt to please the analyst by being normal, it was an escape from the transference. At the same time, it was a means of enjoying the transference, because throughout her elation her analytic hours were filled entirely with facts and phantasies about the boys.
>
> (p. 246)

A Misstep

Wake (2011) argues that 20th-century liberals were blocked by their own internalized prejudices despite their push for liberal public attitudes. In the case of Marian, Thompson was aware of her sexual conflicts and her attempt to please the analyst by "being normal." Being a culturalist, it is surprising that Thompson did not convey to the patient how the pressure of compulsory heterosexuality may have kept her from acknowledging her sexuality. Thompson may have been blocked by her own internalized prejudice, and conflicts about her bisexuality. She did not know what is commonly known now—that suicide is more frequent among homosexual youth (Haas & Drescher, 2014)—if she had known, she might have seen Marian as being more at risk. To her credit, she did not pathologize Marian. She seemed aware but unengaged with the erotic transference Marian communicates in her dreams. Given that homophobia was rampant in America and in psychoanalysis, Thompson may have gone as far as she could.[3]

It is commendable that Thompson chose to write about her struggle with a difficult patient with a tragic ending. Since the treatment ended in suicide, she surely was criticized, and she felt guilty about her role in the outcome. She could have presented another treatment that cast her in a more positive light, but her interest was in the process of inquiry regardless of where it led.

The Use of Identification

In "Identification with the Enemy and Loss of the Sense of Self" (1940b), Thompson theorizes from the case material of six patients, including Marian.

> The child unable to cope with the hostility directed toward him may renounce his own interests for the sake of peace and takes over his parent's attitudes. This may be called identification with the enemy, and one would expect it to be inhibitory to personality development, as are all defense mechanisms.

(p. 38)

Thompson distinguishes between identification and imitation, using the example of what happens when someone lives in a country led by a dictator to make her point.

> An illustration of both identification and imitation can be found in the attitudes of individuals living in countries ruled by dictators where

nonconformity to the current ideologies may be punished by death. Many people under these conditions conform outwardly but keep their own inner counsel.

They think otherwise. On the other hand there are individuals who are actually "converted" to the current ideology through fear. They close their minds to any critical attitude about it. They no longer dare to doubt its rightness. This latter group may be classed with the type of patient reported in this paper. These patients one would suspect are people confronted by unusual danger.

It is not strange, therefore, that the individuals who first attracted the author's attention to the subject were psychotic. Probably the psychotic group does not as a whole fall under this pattern. There is, therefore, no intention to generalize about all psychotic individuals. The aim is rather to describe and understand the implications of one type of object relationship shown especially clearly in some of them.

(p. 38)

Compliance as a Form of Resistance

Thompson introduces another important concept in "'Dutiful Child' Resistance" (sic) (1931). She argues that a compliant child can develop a form of detachment, where outwardly the child appears cooperative, but her compliance is a form of defensive resistance. Drawing on two analytic cases, she explains how the origin of this type of resistance can be found in many patients. In the first case, a 40-something woman suffers from various states of fear. Her symptoms grew worse over a ten-year period.

At the time of beginning analysis she was unable to walk on the street alone, and suffered great anxiety even when accompanied. She was also unable to remain in a house alone—at the same time she felt suffocated when in a room with anyone else, and must have at least one window open, no matter what the temperature.

(p. 425)

The second case is a young man who complained of a lack of interest, ambition, and feelings of despair about life.

He fears that he cannot succeed at anything. Further—when a venture seems to be going smoothly, he has a compulsion to do something in order to fail. He also was a timid child, fearing rough playmates and the usual aggressive boy interests. In any situation of stress he had the tendency to seek the protection of his nurse or mother.

(p. 428)

Thompson points out that neither patient was conscious of any feeling of lack of maternal love—in fact they admired their mother. Thompson does not at first suspect that a "dutiful child" attitude is at work nor that it was the basis of analytic resistance.

These patients behaved very similarly in analysis. From the beginning, the attitude was one of extreme docile cooperation. Everything seemed to go unusually smoothly. A minimum of time was wasted on unessentials; associations ran almost exclusively on childhood material. Every suggestion was accepted without apparent criticism or doubt . . . the analyst was never permitted to be in error, but fantasies were even constructed to prove the correctness of interpretations. However, as time went on two things became apparent one, that, in spite of uncovering an important material, there was no change in symptoms. The patients did not complain of this—they acted rather as if they would like to keep it from the analyst—one fearing that it might discourage her and she would give up on the case. The second significant point was that the analyst seemed to figure almost not at all in the picture. There was seldom any reference to her—and little things which usually irritate, such as lateness or interruptions produced no comment. When this fact was brought to the attention of the first patient, she said that it had never occurred to her to think of the analysts as a person: "You are the doctor—I am paying you to analyze me. I am not so foolish as to expect you to be especially interested in me," etc . . . one is tempted to believe this is an unusually reasonable patient with an attitude based on reality . . . however it was but the cloak of an unusually powerful transference, i.e., the need of the analyst here was so great that no demands must be made which might jeopardize the relation. Both patients within a short time after beginning analysis experienced relief of symptoms during the analytic hour, a relief which could not at that time had been due to insight and must be attributed to transference. Moreover, these patients promptly became much worse whenever analysis was interrupted for a few days as in summer vacations.

These facts forced the conclusion that an affective relationship to the analyst must exist, although the patient was not conscious of it.

(p. 429)

Thompson resolves the clinical problem by bringing the patient's unconscious feelings into the treatment.

In a footnote Thompson maintains, "This was finally brought about by Ferenczi's neo-catharsis method. (A description of this was first given at the International Psychoanalytic Congress at Oxford in 1929.) In the first case, where the method has been tried for only a short period (about two months), there has been little alteration in the "dutiful child" attitude, but in the second case, where the method has been used for nearly a year, there are practically no traces of the "dutiful child" left.

Thompson was most likely drawing from her own psychoanalytic treatment with Ferenczi when she describes what happens when someone grows up feeling unloved and develops a facade of compliance. It becomes critical for the child not to upset the unloving parent. She comes to understand that her compliant patients have no real confidence in her as their analyst. Instead, they feel they must use and manage her by concealing their true feelings.

The use of false feelings kept them out of harm as children now as adults they use the same approach with the analyst. It is as if the patient is saying—"you have no real feelings for me—you are acting the part of a mother—I also will act a part."—"I see through you, but do not be afraid or angry; I will not betray you; in fact, I will play the same game. You pretend your feelings; I will pretend mine."

(p. 432)

Thompson identifies the developmental challenge as not that the patient's mother did not love him, "but that she pretended she did" (p. 432).

It seems apparent that the dutiful child is essentially a reaction to unadmitted insincerity in the individual upon whom the patient is completely dependent for security; that is, it is essentially an imitation of that individual's insincerity and hides the real attitude of the patient.

(p. 433)

Thompson's model of psychoanalysis grew out of her experience in her analysis with Ferenczi. In that analysis, she was recognized, responded to, and was the recipient of his love and tenderness. She argues that patients need a new experience in therapy. Echoing Ferenczi, she finds a restrained analytic attitude can become "an almost perfect reproduction of the deprivations in their childhood relations:"

> In cases when the patient suffered great love deprivation in childhood, it is necessary for the analyst to undertake a kind of adoption that is necessary to give the patient some experience in childhood love before he can realize that he has missed it.
>
> (p. 430)

Both "'Dutiful Child' Resistance" (1931) and "Identification with the Enemy and Loss of the Sense of Self" (1940b) were drafted during her treatment with Ferenczi. In these papers, she allows the reader access to her clinical thinking as she explains how she arrives at an understanding of how to reach her patients and encourage them to be curious about their inner lives. She is attuned to the role she occupies vis-a-vis her patients and their wished-for outcome of what amounts to a balanced internal life.

Detachment

In the essay "Development of Awareness of Transference in a Markedly Detached Personality" (1938b), Thompson not only examines the use of detachment as a defense but in doing so she illustrates the form of transference in the treatment of a detached patient.

> The obstacle encountered in analyzing a narcissistic individual is the problem of obtaining a relationship in which the transference is sufficiently positive to make some form of interpersonal relationship possible. One encounters either a marked overt hostility or a detachment.
>
> (p. 299)

She describes the detached patient as:

> unaware of any personal emotional contact with other human beings. He is an onlooker at life. When it is necessary for him to have a relationship with another human being, he either conducts this relationship

as coldly as if it were an unimportant business transaction, or he goes through the motions of social graciousness or friendliness without having the slightest feelings corresponding to the behavior or, if the detachment is extreme, as in some schizophrenic states, even these efforts at communication may be given up.

(p. 299)

She discusses a five-year analysis with a man who initially showed a "total absence of transference" and who, over time, established an "awareness of its existence." She traces the events in the analytic encounter that she believed touched him.

> First, after being rebuffed by a girl, the patient expected the analyst to disapprove and instead found her supportive of him: "For the first time he became aware that he cared what she thought of him" (p. 306). The second event occurred when the analyst received news of a death of a close friend just before his session. He was "surprised and touched that the analyst dared show her grief unashamed to him. He felt kindly toward her because of this" (p. 306).

Another episode of feeling occurred when

> the patient preceding him had carelessly flung his coat over three hooks instead of one in the closet as if he were perfectly at home. The patient was suddenly consumed with rage when he saw it and felt a strong impulse to fling the other patient's coat on the floor. The intensity of his own reaction surprised him and made him realize that he felt he must never take any liberties, because he still felt very uncertain of the analyst's approval.

(p. 307)

The final disappearance of his detachment came by the same dramatic sudden breaking through of feeling as on the other occasions. The precipitating cause was a mistake on the analyst's part. She was caught napping. The patient was talking of an important childhood experience. The analyst believed it was being told for the first time and indicated her interest in it as new data. The patient became pale, began to sweat and a look of terror came into his face as he said "Do you mean to say you don't remember my mentioning this before, I've talked about it at least three times." This statement was probably true, for subsequent study of the notes has shown that it had been recorded once before. The patient went on to say that probably the analyst never listened to him, that that was why he couldn't get well and how had he been so foolish as to trust his life to such a person. He became physically ill with fever, diarrhea, and vomiting lasting for twenty-four hours. His worst fear had been realized, he was too unimportant even to be listened to, and it mattered to him. He knew now definitely that he cared tremendously for the analyst's approval. But the humiliation was not all on his side—he saw now that she was a bad analyst not only incompetent but "criminally negligent." He realized that whatever doubts he had had of her as a person he had nursed the illusion that she was the most perfect analyst in the world. All of his disillusionment came out with very beneficial results.

(p. 307)

This essay is instructive for the way Thompson illuminates aspects of transference. She shows how discrepancies in the patient's expectations are revealed in analytic work and how the introduction of a new and genuine experience can be transformative.

The Presence of the Analyst

Thompson's essay "Notes on the Psychoanalytic Significance of the Choice of Analyst" (1938c) published in the journal *Psychiatry* five years after the death of Ferenczi, is pivotal. She introduces the concept of reciprocity in the analytic encounter arguing for the mutually influencing role of the analyst and patient.

Any study of the phenomenon that appear in psychoanalysis has its difficulties. The context is prolonged over a long period, meaning often attaches to subtleties that are hard to recapture, and fully convincing explorations have usually to be admitted in the interest of the therapeutic result. There are, however, some published data of observation that can be appraised objectively. Of this information, that pertaining to the analyst's part in the collaboration is the more glaringly inadequate. One seldom finds an account of anything that suggests the differences in personality of various psychoanalysts, or the significant entering of the analyst's personality anywhere in the whole protracted process. Many analysts, however, must have failed with some patient who did better elsewhere; must have carried to completion some patients who had failed with a preceding analyst. Moreover, every psychoanalysis has a beginning, and patients often exercise what is called choice in selecting the person with whom they will undertake the work.

(p. 205)

Here Thompson is announcing a sea change in the practice of psychoanalysis. She situates the analyst and their attitudes as equally important to the analysis as those of the patient's. This ushers in a new, American psychoanalysis with a newly developing tradition, interpersonal psychoanalysis. The message in Thompson's essay is a non-Freudian view of human relationships and a view of the analytic encounter that integrates the social sciences.

An individual has some personal reaction to every one with whom he comes in close contact and an analyst presumably is no exception in this respect. The fact, he might be expected to have some very definite feelings about someone who he expects to see daily for many months, perhaps years. While material is easily available on that rational and irrational or transference attitudes of patients, since they are important things to be investigated in every analysis, it is more difficult to observe the attitudes of the analyst and evaluate their influences on the analysis.

(p. 206)

As Ferenczi's direct clinical descendent, Thompson is stating that the field of inquiry in psychoanalysis is broader than that of the patient's internal world; it includes the analyst and is interactional. She does not begin where Ferenczi left off by quoting him or his teachings, as she could quickly have done by referencing "The Elasticity of Psychoanalytic Technique" (1928), an essay Rachman (1997) notes that offers a two-person view of the analytic relationship. Instead, she uses her own individually American voice as she steers psychoanalysis into the mainstream of American empiricism. She talks about objectivity, observation, and data. Her audience—the social scientists Sullivan (1938) has assembled for his journal—is interdisciplinary. It includes sociologists, anthropologists, political scientists, physicians, and psychologists, as well as psychoanalysts. Thompson, the spokesperson for this new psychoanalysis, although an admittedly reserved person, is independent with an educational background grounded in distinctly American philosophies.

This essay is startling with its ability to go against prevailing authorities and state her ideas clearly and without hesitation. It is important to note that she does this without resorting to criticism or blame. Waugaman (2016) observes that Thompson presents her ideas without the need to dismiss those who hold different opinions. That, along with integrity, is one of her many inspiring leadership strengths. Roger Frie and Pascal Sauvayre (2022) point to the interdisciplinary foundations of interpersonal psychoanalysis fostered in this boundary-breaking volume of the journal *Psychiatry*.[4]

Thompson begins by introducing her work in a manner that can sound as if she is diminishing its own importance: "This essay," she writes, "can be little more than a preliminary communication" (p. 205). She proceeds to take her time to accomplish the exceptional task of explaining something that occurs in each analysis—the selection of the analyst. She provides detailed examples of the permutations and possible complications involved in that important decision.

Waugaman (2016) suggests that Thompson's work goes unacknowledged because she offers balanced opinions that don't grab the attention in the manner that analysts who promote more extreme positions or make it their business to draw attention to their work. Some writers, he suggests, promote their ideas by minimizing the importance of competing authors. Thompson is not interested in self-promotion or fame. In contrast, she is interested in the promotion of ideas. She approaches her work as a researcher/scientist, posing questions, and generating hypotheses. The essay almost reads like a research paper. She states her questions clearly: "(1) What role does the analyst as an individual existing in reality play in the analytic situation? (2) Do individual variations in the analyst have important effects for good or bad on the course of the analysis?" (1938c, p. 205). That is one reason why she qualifies her work with words that minimize rather than aggrandize. Her form of American psychoanalysis has puritan roots—principled, practical, and unadorned. There are no grand pronouncements or empty flattery. She is a scientist at work with a focus on discovery. Penning cautious introductory sentences, she directs attention to the analyst's role as a whole person interacting with the patient, engaging their entire personality to do the work.

She assumes each analyst is sufficiently analyzed and competent. She accepts that a well-analyzed analyst is not infallible but maintains self-observation and self-criticism. She turns to the literature, citing findings of patients' attitudes about their reactions to the analyst and transference phenomenon. She sees flaws in the published data that presents the analyst as either "a fountain of completely detached wisdom in no way affected personally by anything which goes on" or as someone who "puts ideas into the patient's head which he then analyzes out" with none of it related to the patient's life but closer to the "fantasy in the mind of the analyst" (p. 206).

Thompson dismisses these attitudes as untrue. She maintains that emphasizing the need for the analyst to be emotionally detached from the problems of the patient reduces the analyst to a "zero." She gives what she calls a "crude example."

> If the analyst really has no convictions on the question of stealing, can he help the patient to understand and accept the attitude of society in which the patient must live, about stealing?
>
> (p. 206)

This article appeared in *Psychiatry*, the journal that was Sullivan's brainchild. As founding editor, he insisted that the name of his new journal not include the term "psychoanalysis." He wanted to emphasize that the journal would be exploring the spaces between psychiatry, psychoanalysis, the social sciences, and biology. Indeed, the journal's mission statement clarifies that although "psychiatry" is in its title, it is intended for "all serious students of human living in any of its aspects" (William Alanson White Institute, 1938, p. ii).[5] Included in the first volume is Ruth Benedict's (1938) essay on the strength of cultural conditioning, where she posits:

> It is a fact of nature that the child becomes a man, the way in which this transition is effected varies from one society to another, and no one of these particular cultural bridges should be regarded as the "natural" path to maturity.
>
> (p. 161)

Reciprocal Interpersonal

As in other places in her writing, Thompson draws from her own experience and provides examples that sound autobiographical. For example:

> Every so often one finds in reading the report of a detailed case analysis that at a certain point something in reality happens in a session that

convinces the patients of the human qualities of the analyst e.g. some reaction to bad news received over the phone during the patient's hour . . . I, myself, reported the reaction of a schizophrenic patient to my grief at the death of Ferenczi. This convinced him as nothing else had that I was not a cold, aloof, indifferent person, as the rest of his world had been.

(pp. 206, 207)

Green (1964b) gives a similar account:

One day a patient was in consultation with Thompson when the phone rang. She picked up the receiver, listened to it and then hung up, saying to herself and perhaps the patient, "That bitch? That nurse Henry's got says he has cancer of the lung. He has nothing of the sort!"

(p. 371)

The patient may have been Green himself. How else would he have been able to report the event verbatim?

Thompson (1938c) asks:

Is this discovery of the human reaction of the analyst only occasionally of therapeutic value? May it not be that some such knowledge is always essential in the cure of the patient? Isn't being with a detached analyst a replication of a parental detachment that brought the patient into treatment in the first place?

(p. 206)

Always in a conversation with her reader, she asks and answers: "Specifically, what do people want in an analyst? They want most of all someone in whom they can have confidence, someone who makes them feel less afraid, and who they can believe knows how to cure them" (p. 206). She wisely explains that assessing those qualities is next to impossible. No one can really assess an analyst's work, and while training and reputation are important, they don't enter into the assessment in a rational way. The person's reaction to the age of the analyst, as well as cultural background, sex, and personality, is only partially objective. Various other feelings—like strength or hostility on the part of themselves or the analyst—are the subjective ingredients that go into the feeling of trust and confidence: "Irrational or transference factors figure in these feelings as well as reality; that is a patient chooses in the same way that he falls in love, on the basis of his own life patterns" (p. 206). Many people seek out in an analyst a person with whom they feel "most capable of having an intense emotional relationship" (p. 206); undoubtedly that is a familiar personality with whom they tend to have attachments, like a parental figure or the opposite kind of personality or opposite sex of analyst, hoping to avoid those complicated life problems.

Thompson gives clear, persuasive examples in her discussion of the fit between patients and analysts. One in particular may again be autobiographical. She describes a woman who meets an analyst socially; in the course of the evening's conversation, he suggests she come into treatment with him. "Her reaction was fear but she realized that she needed analysis, that he would probably accept her for a fee which she could pay, and finally she felt irresistibly attracted to the situation" (p. 214). This could be a reference to her analytic work with her first therapist, Joseph "Snake" Thompson (see Volume 1). She goes on to describe how

> Analysis was begun, fear continued, sleeplessness developed, difficulty in working appeared, and the patient finally lost her job. The analyst repeatedly urged the patient to seek the sources of her fear of him in her fear of her father—to no avail. The difficulty lay in the analyst. There was in him some tendency to get women away from other men and make them entirely dependent on him. The patient in question had a neurotic attachment to her employer [perhaps this is Adolf Meyer] which was reciprocated by the employer, who also had a neurotic need for power. When this situation began to be analyzed, the analyst's jealousy reinforced the patient's own tendency to make indirect aggressions of a serious nature against her employer with disastrous consequences. Although the patient continued in analysis for some months after the loss of her position, she made no further progress, having lost confidence in the analyst on a reality basis. Later her analysis was successfully completed by another [Sándor Ferenczi].
>
> (p. 214)

Recall that Clara Thompson met Joseph Thompson at a social gathering and went into treatment with him at his suggestion. Feeling Meyer's pressure to terminate her analysis with Joseph Thompson, she resigned (see Volume 1). Like the patient, Thompson also found her first treatment to be of little use, and she later had a successful analysis with Ferenczi. She clearly used her own life experience to add clarity to her clinical examples. She observes that "many analyses fail because a masochistic patient with unconscious genius finds the analyst whose specific liabilities are especially bad for them and hurl themselves to their destruction" (p. 213). It may be that she did hurl herself at Joseph Thompson.

Waugaman (2016) notes how Thompson was ahead of her time in her analysis of certain high-risk analytic dyads. She identifies risk factors for boundary violations: "Some bad analytic situations [sic] occur when the analyst is anxious about a physically illness; or is facing the illness or death of a loved one; or is under financial strain" (p. 16). Her observation has become accepted and discussed widely in the literature (see Gabbard, 2016).

Thompson (1940b) argues that identification is a form of object relationship found in everyone. She sees these identifications primarily as expressions of positive feelings but identification with the aggressor as an ego defense can also occur, as Anna Freud observed. The child feels equal to the threatening authority. But Anna Freud did not account for "what may happen within the child's own personality when the identification is maintained over a long period of time" (p. 36). Thompson clarifies:

> A surrender of part of his own interests. He has taken into himself an ideology not because he admires it or believes in it, but chiefly for protective purposes. The enemy he feared from the outside has so to speak reappeared inside himself. Toward this incorporated imago the young child has greater difficulty in developing a critical attitude toward the friendly one because any attempt to reject it later tends to rouse the same fear which caused its being accepted in the first place.
>
> (Thompson, 1940b, pp. 37–38)

By placing identification within a "normal" paradigm, she says,

> We all know the many ways in which parents are inimical to their children's personalities. . . . One of the most potent of these is the chronic attitude of disapproval. The child unable to cope with the hostility directed toward him may renounce his own interests for the sake of peace and take over his parents' attitudes. This may be called identification with

the enemy, and one would expect it to be inhibitory to personality development, as are all defense mechanisms.

(p. 38)

Identifying through fear may end up as the only means of maintaining object relationships. The individual goes on to make only "hostile" identifications, never living his own life:

> In time he does not know what his own life might be if he were suddenly relapsed and allowed to live it. Moreover, the hostile forces do not live at peace with each other within him; he must now be like one person and now like another and if he has to be like both at once he is in a quandary.
>
> (p. 38)

Love and Re-Living

Ferenczi advocated a departure from the analyst as cool and detached to empathic and loving. He believed "that the patient is ill because he has not been loved, and that he needs from the analyst the positive experience of acceptance, that is, love. This could not be given by a mirror" (Thompson, 1943b, p. 64).

Izette de Forest another analysand of Ferenczi became a life-long friend and colleague of Thompson. In 1942, de Forest published an essay *The Therapeutic Technique of Sándor Ferenczi* where she agreed with her analyst, who she saw as possessing "personal gifts" including a "sensitivity to human suffering" and "creativity." According to de Forest, Ferenczi believed a neurosis developed under the following circumstances:

> there must have actually occurred in childhood . . . (1) a traumatic experience of great intensity, necessitating immediate repression; (2) a sequence of less intense traumatic experiences, which may or may not be wholly repressed; (3) a constant exposure to highly emotional reactions, either sadistic or masochistic, of one or more adults, the memory of which is not entirely repressed. These three types of experience are inevitably of a sexual nature Ferenczi hesitated to assert.
>
> (p. 121)

To defend against these experiences, the child uses "some degree of repression, and then develops a system of "defense mechanism" to guard against "an ever growing anxiety" (p. 120).

De Forest continues that Ferenczi believed the therapeutic process should center:

> dynamically around the mutual relationship of the analyst and patient . . . the analyst's aim is to assist the patient to penetrate through the repressed and distorted experience of his life to the traumatic occurrence or sequence of occurrences which are at the root of the neurosis; then to aid him to face dramatically the trauma or traumatic series by re-living it emotionally, not in its original setting but as an actual part of the analytic situation. The ultimate benefit of having emotionally re-experienced these early crucial moments of his life in an adult environment in which he is protected by the presence and aid of his devoted analyst lies in the transformation of his fear of the overpowering passions within him into a new valuation of them as powerful assets. . . . All that creates the atmosphere of parent and child being intimately together helps to maintain the dynamic relation that Ferenczi considered necessary. . . . Constant effort must be made by the analyst to pull the patient's emotional reactions back into the analytic setting, always brining the analyst into the center by relation all associations and attention on to himself.
>
> (pp. 120–121)

Thompson (1943b) responded to de Forest's essay with, *The Therapeutic Technique of Sándor Ferenczi: A Comment.* She explains that she too largely made use of Ferenczi's techniques and agreed with de Forest's account of his work. However, she differed from Ferenczi and "discarded" a few of his ideas. First, she thought inducing a regression through an intense re-living of an experience could be risky to the patient. Second, she felt that love was a complicated emotion that could be used by patients in ways Ferenczi and de Forest did not consider. "Ferenczi," Thompson argues, "tended to confuse the idea that the patient must be given all the love he needs with the idea he must be given all the love he demands" (p. 65). Thompson closes her comments agreeing with de Forest on the importance of Ferenczi's emphasis on the significance of the real personality of the analyst in the total situation.

> I believe it plays a part in the patient's cure. I also agree that the analyst must give the patient the 'love' he needs if he is to have enough security to proceed. That this loving of the patient must be spontaneous and disinterested, i.e. not growing out of any need of the analyst's, goes without saying. I am sure that I cannot endorse the lengths to which Ferenczi went in this matter. I feel that Mrs. de Forest [Izette de Forest was not a physician] also differs from me somewhat here. I have the impression she feels that more definite assertions of liking are necessary than I have found to be the case. However, my real difference with her and Ferenczi is about the therapeutic value of building up tension deliberately in order to increase the dramatic tone of the analysis. I do not deny that at times this may have a therapeutic effect, but, in general, I believe it not only has no therapeutic value but actually increases the patient's hazards.
>
> (pp. 65–66)

Later de Forest published the book *The Leaven of Love: A Development of the Psychoanalytic Theory and Technique of Sándor Ferenczi* (1954), where she again described Ferenczi's approach to therapy, providing clinical examples from her own work. Erich Fromm wrote a review of *The Leaven of Love* (NYTimes, 1955)[6] He also notes that "Ferenczi himself never did record these ideas systematically." He points out that Ferenczi came to believe that the gift of therapeutic love had indispensable healing power.

> In personal discussions with Mrs. De Forest, Ferenczi formulated his new principle in this way: Psychoanalytic 'cure' is in direct proportion to the cherishing love given by the psychoanalyst to the patient: the love which the psychoneurotic patient *needs*.
>
> (p. 98)

Soon after Ferenczi's death de Forest, like Clara Thompson, turned to Erich Fromm for another analysis.

Race, Sex, and Gender

Thompson confronted her own racist, sexist, and homophobic ideas in her essays. She did not have the benefit of critical race theory to guide her. Rather she relied on a set of values and beliefs in fairness and equality that shaped her early life. There are progressive steps as well as flaws and contradictions in her attempts to theorize. An in-depth look reveals the incongruities, but it also demonstrates her fairness. In "Dynamics of Hostility" (1959a), she speaks of race in a way that was rare for psychoanalysis:

> If one lives constantly in an unfriendly environment, as in the case of the American Negro, it is normal to show a chronic hostility toward one's persecutors. These, I believe cannot be considered destructive drives; they are a part of man's expression of his right and wish to live.
>
> (pp. 10–11)

Diving deeper, she takes a more conservative turn:

> However, all of these emotions can become expressions of irrational or pathological attitudes, and it is this aspect which is the concern of the psychoanalyst. When the degree of expression of anger, rage, hate, or hostility is out of all proportion to the apparent immediate inciting cause, we are dealing with something which goes beyond immediate self-preservation; in fact, it is often self-destructive. However, even irrational behavior usually has an understandable beginning.
>
> Just as normal hostility has its origin in justifiable fear of real danger, irrational hostility has its origin in anxiety.
>
> (p. 11)

Thompson flips back and forth between consciously acknowledging the inequality and hostility shown to people of color in this country along with the justifiable anger that comes with that exploitation. She then reverts to what she knows best—psychiatric and psychoanalytic theories that tend to pathologize individual feelings rather than turn a light on the society where they are embedded. Had she recognized systemic oppression as the "concern of the psychoanalyst," she would have been an activist.

In "An Introduction to Minor Maladjustments" (1959c), she again entered into an uncommon clinical discussion of race relations, naming a cultural "hazard" present in society and identified in Fromm's *The Sane Society*. She explains the trap as

> a conflict between the "true" convictions of the individual and expediency, in terms of acceptance by others. If one has subscribed to the importance of being successful, being what is expected of him with the hope of winning power, it is very disrupting to personal integrity and even to sanity if the price of this means denial of valued basic principles. An example is the following: a man believing in the rights of Negros is in a position of authority in a Southern state. He can belligerently espouse the cause of Negros and probably, thereby, lose whatever status he has. He thinks maybe he should take a middle-of -the- road course— but then he becomes confused. Is he deciding upon his course because it will produce the best results in the long run, or is he influenced by his personal ambition to be accepted in win a more impressive position in the community? The state of conflict between the two ideas develops, so that he no longer is able to decide what is best for the cause of the Negros, the cause to which he thought he was dedicated. What got in the way was his marketing need for personal success, and his final choice was determined by his personal ambition. But some part of him could not accept his decision, and presently he consulted a psychiatrist because of depression and suicidal thoughts. In stating his problem, he said "I cannot understand why I am so unhappy. So far I have accomplished everything I set out to do, and it looks as if I would get the next position I am seeking." Because he was a person unusually honest with himself, the cause of his unhappiness soon was made clear to him. The issue here is not whether the more effective course is to be radical or middle of the road, but the fact that the need to be successful personally was obscuring his judgment. This man might have gone on to the end of his days, pursuing his personal ambitions without realizing their marketing character, if he had not come into conflict with the prejudices of his community, which forced him to face his values.
>
> (p. 243)

She explains,

> An important thing to remember in considering the people described in this chapter is that the obviously neurotic person suffers from his

failure to adapt, but these people I am discussing suffer from the compromises they have made in order to adapt.

(p. 244)

She adds that both sets of individuals suffer from their need for approval.

Public Life Private Life

More can be gleaned about Thompson by looking beyond her expressed public attitudes on race by a closer examination of her private life. There we find inconsistencies. She had a significant and continuing relationship with Lillie Fisher, an African American woman who worked in Thompson's home for 30 years.

Fisher took care of Thompson's household and looked after her as well. Silverberg (1959), a colleague of Thompson's, recalls Fisher's

> southern cooking and her utter loyalty to Thompson. Her loyalty sometimes took the form of petulant scolding, which Clara bore with great equanimity. Her relationship with Lilly, endured throughout nearly her entire life.
>
> (Silverberg, 1959, p. 3)

Fisher was only ten years older than Thompson but seems to have been experienced as a nurturing maternal figure. The 1930 US Census lists Fischer as a widow who had married at age 28. She was close to her own sister, Lottie Taylor of Baltimore. She had no schooling and was a cook. In 1930, she is listed as living as a boarder with her sister Lottie and her husband, Jas-L-Taylor. Thompson's feelings for Fisher are poignantly expressed in her letter to Fromm on March 11, 1956 (housed in the Erich Fromm archive, Tubingen):

> As for the rest of me—Lillie left me today. For the first time in many years I am alone in the big world. No mother. Honestly my heart ached more for her than for me. She had dedicated her life to me. I am all that she has. I shall be kind to her always. I owe her a great deal. Why do parents always have to be hurt?

Thompson's last will and testament stated, "I give to Lillie Fisher who was my maid for thirty years my account in the state mutual building association of Baltimore; and . . . to her my clothing." The money was a sign of her love, gratitude, and respect. Lillie Fisher was residing at 2208 Druid Hill Road, Baltimore when Thompson died. This address is listed as a 1920's townhouse in one of Baltimore's earliest African American middle-class neighborhoods. Following her retirement, Fisher returned to her community and rejoined her family. Her obituary reads that Lillie was the beloved sister of Lottie Taylor and was surrounded by many relatives and friends. The discrepancy between Thompson's expression of sorrow over Fisher being alone and what appears to be the reality of Fisher's life with her family in retirement is striking. Various questions arise about the nature of their relationship.

On Not Knowing

Thompson and Fisher both knew and did not know each other. One wonders how Fisher felt about "mothering" Thompson. There seems to be confusion over who was caring for whom in their relationship speaking to the complexity in their roles.[7]

Thompson's mother was harsh and cold. She must have welcomed the warmth and care Fisher offered. But did their relationship fall victim to an American stereotype—Fisher, a black woman, working for Thompson, a white woman, in the role of maid/mother. (McElya, 2007; Wallace-Sanders, 2008). Perry (1982) discusses Thompson's move to Baltimore and Fisher's employment in language that suggests prevailing racist attitudes: "She acquired a black live-in housekeeper" (p. 209). "Acquired" is the tell.

Yet, Thompson's early upbringing instilled in her a set of ideals that led her to value fairness, she was less judgmental than her counterparts and less conventional, but she was still a white woman of privilege.[8] Thompson and Fisher somehow held the complications of their power differentials in their relationship over decades.[9]

To Thompson's credit, in, "*Changing Concepts of Homosexuality in Psychoanalysis*" (1947), she also took up the construct and the cultural attitudes toward homosexuality in a virulently anti-homosexual post-war America. At the time her ideas were bold. She maintained that "various personality problems may find partial solution in a homosexual symptom, but nothing has been shown as specifically producing homosexuality" (p. 188).

We can imagine her friendships with Sullivan and Ruth Benedict influenced her ideas on homosexuality, yet together their ideas were all contained within 20th-century language of sexuality and identity.

> People who for reasons external to their own personality find their choice of love object limited to their own sex may be said to be "normal homosexuals," in the sense that they utilized the best type of interpersonal relationship available to them. These people are not the problem of psychopathology.
>
> (Thompson, 1947, p. 186)

Thompson was also practical when it came to homosexuality. Wake (2011) describes how Thompson asked help from Sullivan to get her patient out of the army. Thompson believed that "it would be disastrous [for the patient] to go in the army." She asked Sullivan to use his influence and get the patient a rejection without diagnosing him as homosexual (p. 168). She was aware of what a diagnosis would mean to the patient and what being gay in the army would do to his well-being.

Twentieth-Century Liberalism: Successes and Failures

Sullivan, Thompson, and their colleagues were a small group of liberals in a sea of conservatives. Their attempts at promoting their liberal attitudes fell far short of their aspirations. Even though the 20th-century social scientists turned away from the 19th-century codification of people as immature, pathological, and diseased toward a more-alike-than-different attitude in their public positions; privately they held attitudes that remained hostile and unaccepting (Wake, 2011). In some cases, although gay themselves, they held anti-homosexual or racist attitudes. Their internalized homophobia and racism remained unexamined. In some cases, the opposite was also true, that is, their private attitudes were liberal, while public personas were conservative. This "gap," argues Wake, prevented mainstream public activism and shored up homophobic and racist policies.

While Sullivan held progressive liberal views on race, unconsciously he may have used race as a way to distance himself from the injustices he experienced as a gay man (Wake, p. 112). Sullivan worked closely with the American scholar E. Franklin Frazier, a black sociologist. He helped

Frazier get his research funded. Frazier's dissertation, "The Negro Family in the United States" (1939), examined the historical forces that influenced African American families. He was the first black scholar to study and write about the African American experience and Sullivan was his research consultant. In the process of their work together, Sullivan interviewed about 20 "African American youths," noting that he did not find any typical Negro characteristics among his informants.[10]

> At the same time, Sullivan said, "white Americans must 'cultivate a humanistic rather than a paternalistic attitude' to blacks" (p. 112). But in private, he suggested that "his white male friend sleep with black women to become free sexually" (p. 147), a clear objectification of black women. He also suggested to his patient's brother that the patient might improve enough under proper treatment to live outside a hospital, maybe on a small farm with a black man to look after him, someone he could scream at and even hit who wouldn't hurt him and would care for him whatever he did.
>
> (p. 147)

Sullivan, Thompson, and others in this cohort struggled to escape cultural biases, making small steps in that direction. Were they thwarted by their unexamined internalized attitudes? Wake warns that those who seek to destroy progressive politics seek out those cracks in their positions and exploit them. A lesson we can learn from these 20th-century liberals is to be mindful that our publicly expressed aspirations for change might be thwarted if we do not address our privately internalized assumptions.[11]

Creating the Interpersonal Tradition

Four additional essays essential to the discussion of Thompson's opus are: "Transference as a Therapeutic Instrument" (1945); "Countertransference" (1952); "Transference and Character Analysis" (1953); and "Concepts of Self in Interpersonal Theory" (1958a), each expressing Thompson's ideas about clinical psychoanalytic practice. In each, the mutually interactive quality of analysis—and with it, the irrational elements that can make their way into the consulting room—as well as the real and positive feelings that develop between patient and analyst are addressed. Transference, she argues, "was not created by psychoanalysis" (Thompson, 1954, p. 273).

There have always been irrational elements in every human relationship, and they are prone to show up in attitudes "where one of the two people is in a position of authority in relation to the other" (p. 274). She finds Freud's views on transference simpler than the complicated defenses she observes.

> Increased knowledge of character structure has shown that transference is a much more complicated mechanism and includes more attitudes than the simple positive and negative ones first described.
>
> (p. 274)

Transference as a Therapeutic Instrument was given as a paper on April 27, 1945, at a meeting of the American Psychopathological Association, and published that year in *Psychiatry*. In that essay, Thompson extends Ferenczi's notion that there are real positive and negative feelings held by the patient and analyst that are not necessarily transference. Kay (2014), commenting on Thompson's paper, points to how her observations would later become what we call a working alliance. (p. 6) Providing some helpful examples, Kay explains,

> To explicate this point more concretely in my teaching to residents, I might refer to the myth of the analyst as blank screen that categorizes all feelings by the patient as distortions placed onto the analyst. In other words, this would constitute a one-person model of treatment. This notion, of course, is a caricature of what transpires in analysis but is illustrative of a position that the analyst's contributions to the dyad, be it his demeanor, personality, or speech, are somehow less significant than that of the patient's. Thompson, then, is foreshadowing what will evolve from self-psychology and relational/intersubjective psychoanalysis. The latter argues that there can be no effective treatment without the appreciation that the contributions of the analyst/therapist are as important as those of the patient and that the treatment experience is a co-creation by the patient and analyst. Simply, Thompson urges to move beyond blaming the patient and to appreciate the role of the analyst's personality and capacity to evoke certain feelings in the patient that determine his or her unconscious response based on earlier developmental experiences.
>
> (pp. 6–7)

Countertransference

In her essay "Countertransference" (1952), Thompson takes up the feelings of the analyst, offering the following clinical vignette,

> on one occasion I found myself getting annoyed with a patient who frequently used the wrong form of the pronoun after a preposition. He would say, "from Frank and I." Here I am sure the annoyance was my problem and not his, i.e., it was counter-transference. On the other hand, if one finds oneself getting annoyed at a patient who consistently finds it hard to leave, this, can be an indication that something is wrong, and the matter should be more thoroughly discussed. Whatever is going on in the patient is not clear to him or to the analyst. It is very important to distinguish between these two motives . . . in the first case the analyst must look into his own difficulties. In the second situation, he must investigate the motives of the patient. . . . It is clear that not all feelings experienced by the analyst in relation to his patient are in a strictly technical sense, countertransference. Countertransference proper should be carefully defined as the transference of irrational aspects of the analyst's personality to the relationship with his patient. This invariably makes for difficulties, and it is in order to eliminate as much of this as possible that the personal analysis of the analyst is required. The analyst . . . should be as free from anxiety and defensive attitudes as it is humanly possible to be . . . because he is human he will sometimes be tired or ill. Tragedies may happen in his life all of these things are likely to have some repercussion on his relationship with the patient. Tiredness may merely lower his efficiency in observing or it may increase his irritability so that he may lose patience at some difficult moment. Illness or a personal tragedy adds the complicating factor of worry or preoccupation with oneself. This may lead to such thoughts on the part of the analyst as "I am worse off than the patient. What is he complaining about?"
>
> (p. 205)

Thompson provides examples to illustrate her clinical points. She was a talented teacher and supervisor. She explores how the analyst's supervisor can have an impact on the analyst's work with patients. She ends the essay advising, "[Y]ou may end by learning something new about yourself if you really keep your ear tuned to trying to understand what is going on between you and the patient" (p. 211).

"Transference and Character Analysis" (1953)

A decade after her first essay on transference, Thompson takes up the subject again in "Transference and Character Analysis" (1953). This time, she argues that psychoanalysis has been slow to examine the similarities of transference and character resistance.

> Freud's first simple formulation was that the patient relived in analysis his feelings towards his parents at the Oedipus period. These attitudes were seen as irrational in that they did not make sense when applied to the relationship to the physician. Moreover, they seemed to serve as an obstacle to the progress of the analysis. When all was going smoothly there would suddenly have to be time out while the patient picked a fight or engaged in some other emotional reaction to the analyst. . . . By reliving the emotions of the past the meaning of these earlier experiences became clear. All of this made sense and for many years there was little modification of the early theory, but around 1920 Freud made some new revolutionary discoveries, one of which was the repetition compulsion. . . . Freud concluded that transference was a typical example of the repetition compulsion. In transference were repeated automatically feelings and reactions of earlier periods even when those experiences were unpleasant. . . . Rank and Ferenczi discovered the importance in the picture of the analyst in his own right—thus transference became more precisely defined as only the irrational attitudes felt and expressed toward the analyst. At this point, Rank and Ferenczi as well as Sullivan were beginning to define the analytical situation as an *inter-personal process* (italics added) although this was not explicitly so stated. . . . All these discoveries contributed significantly to the working out of a method of character analysis, and work around this has come to be known as ego psychology . . . this term is used to describe the largely unconscious defensive activities of the ego in carrying out its function of making the individual acceptable to his environment.
>
> (pp. 260–262)

Thompson describes Sullivan's concepts filtered through her own lens, interweaving her ideas without fanfare. She does not take credit.

The Self

Thompson's essay *Concepts of Self in Interpersonal Theory* (1958a) was originally given as a talk.[12] In it, she makes a radical departure from Freud's libidinal metapsychology as she presents the views of the by-then-deceased Sullivan (he died in 1949) with, as she says, "comments, criticisms and conclusions of my own" (Unpublished paper, WAW Archive).

She proceeds to take up Sullivan's controversial concept of the self, arguing it was inconsistent. On the one hand, Sullivan sees the self as "a product of the dynamic forces of interaction with others, and on the other hand "that it is a subject outside of his sphere of interest and, therefore no concern of his" (p. 5). Sullivan thought "all that one can know positively about another person is what can be observed in his relationship to one's self and others. He limited his theory to what goes on between people while claiming "this is not the whole story of human personality" (p. 5).

Thompson reiterates that for Sullivan "the human personality" is formed by "interactions with others."

> The baby is born without a sense of self. It is generally agreed that during the first weeks of life, the infant has no way of distinguishing himself from his mother, or the mothering one.
>
> (p. 6)

Thompson shows her willingness to use a more gender-free language as she speaks of the "mothering one" moving into Sullivan's theory of development.

> As the baby gradually becomes aware of himself as an entity separate from the mother, he begins to notice that he seems to have some control over at least some of the moods of the mother. She is angry when he does some things and pleasant when he does others. The desire to please her thus grows out of his own desire to feel comfortable. . . . Discovery of a part of the universe over which he has control, and which in time becomes known as "my body," Sullivan suggested has much to do with firmly entrenched feelings of an independent, autonomous entity, which gives what he has called, "the delusion of unique individuality."
>
> (pp. 6–7)

Thompson explains Sullivan's ideas by providing her own examples:

> As the developing personality unfolds, the child begins to think of the
> sum total of behavior as "me." Then he begins to learn that aspects of "my
> body" and "me" at times meet with forbidding attitudes. Since the human
> infant needs tenderness, and approval for growth and survival, he begins
> to sacrifice parts of the "me," which are creating difficulty and, in his
> primitive thinking, he entertains the idea of a "good me" and a "bad me."
>
> (p. 9)

Digging deeper she discusses "good me," "bad me," and "not me." Sullivan's concept of the self is based on the avoidance of anxiety in interaction
with the self- systems of others. She explains that the basic assumption is
that human beings have a basic need for closeness and only in that closeness can one feel secure.

> This need for security is fully as insistent and important as the need for
> satisfaction of hunger, thirst, sex, etc. In fact, in some ways, it is more
> insistent. . . . Man, therefore, needs to be related to others, not only for
> physical security, but, lacking strong innate instinct patterns, he needs
> association with others in order to learn how to live. This learning how
> to live through example, imitation, acceptance, and punishment cre-
> ates the self-system. If the rules of acceptance and punishment are very
> rigid, that is if failure to conform is very severely punished, the self-
> system will be very rigid, and any experimental attempts to behave
> differently from the prescribed pattern will produce extreme anxiety,
> so that the attempt is usually abandoned. . . . Let me repeat here, this
> personality has been formed to a great extent through reactions to
> approval and disapproval on the part of significant people, and these
> significant people have, therefore, produced a product which is usually
> easily recognized as belonging to a particular culture. In fact, it may be
> possible to observe that this person is a product of a particular group in
> a particular culture, and as every psychoanalyst can testify, the marks
> of the impact of the particular parents are also evident. . . . This means
> that many of the attitudes of the others are incorporated as if they were
> established facts, modifications of impulses are developed to avoid dis-
> approval, and being accepted by the important others is the goal.
>
> (Thompson, 1958a, pp. 10–11)

Thompson separates herself from Sullivan noting that Sullivan believed "that the self-system tends to be relatively rigid and not easily modifiable by experience."

> In my opinion, he cannot have meant that the total self is relatively rigid. There seem to be all degrees of flexibility in it. Characteristics which have never encountered either strong approval or disapproval may change easily under the impact of new circumstances or even from further growth within.
>
> (p. 12)

She argues further that, for some people, there are disturbances that

> produce only mild anxiety, and may be fairly easily changed; but most people have a more-or-less extensive rigid portion, which has been developed in response to intense threat of anxiety.
>
> (p. 12)

Here she shows more flexibility than Sullivan. She maintains that his concept of dissociation addressed the way the self manages potentialities and behavior that are unacceptable in a particular culture, group, or family. Thompson understands Sullivan's concept of anxiety as an amplification of Freud's theory of anxiety without the concept of libido. She writes,

> Thus, I do not believe the self, in interpersonal theory, is entirely the product of the attempt to avoid anxiety, but it is nevertheless a product of the society in which it develops. Every society offers certain types of opportunity to the young. It is not so much that it always forbids other opportunity, although "forbidding" accounts for some nondevelopment, . . . The individual is truly a product of his culture as brought to him, first through his parents and later through his other life opportunities. Only rarely does there occur a maverick, one whose life experiences somehow made him a rebel rather than a conformist. But even then, the degree of his deviation is not permitted to be unlimited. Beyond a certain point society forbids his deviation, and few can survive that degree of disapproval.
>
> (p. 13)

Thompson's concept of self is more flexible and more nuanced, influenced by a variety of circumstances,

> Under circumstances of great stress or temptation, unaccepta-
> ble aspects may erupt in spite of the disapproval of the significant
> people . . . we all do things at times of which we are ashamed and of
> which we may have previously thought we were incapable; but at least
> if we do not deny to ourselves that we have done it, we may be strong
> enough to stand the anxiety of keeping it in consciousness. . . . Alter-
> ing the self also occurs when the significant people in our lives change
> and, in adapting to the new situation, certain characteristics may be
> pushed aside and others allowed to emerge . . . new circumstances fur-
> nish new stimuli . . . this change can be in a constructive or destructive
> direction . . . when change results in a constructive expansion of the
> self in the course of weakening the rigidity of the self-system . . . the
> person on finds himself in a less threatening environment than he had
> previously experienced. Hitherto undeveloped potentialities are dis-
> covered and encouraged, resulting in a fuller, more fruitful life. Such
> is the change to be observed during the analytic process. We say "he is
> discovering himself" meaning that the cramping circumstances of his
> earlier life are being removed and his capabilities are becoming more
> apparent. Is he, as we are fond of saying discovering his true self?
>
> (pp. 13–14)

Thompson explains that Sullivan rejected the idea of a unique individual. He saw no "existence of a self, separate from the person created by his culture" (p. 15). On the other hand, for Thompson, potentiality is important. While Sullivan believed,

> a person who has never known love or tenderness as a small child is
> permanently incapable of recognizing or experiencing it in later years.
>
> (p. 15)

She argues instead that if we believe,

> there is somewhere in us a true self apart from cultural experience,
> we would have to assume, I think, that potentiality for love resides in

everyone, and can, therefore, be developed at any time, contrary to Sullivan's belief.

(p. 15)

Thompson had argued like Sullivan that a person who was not loved as a child cannot make use of love even when offered it as an adult. She too is inconsistent—or, perhaps, she changed her mind over time.

She concludes that Sullivan's theory

> leaves no place for including undeveloped potentialities within the self. Unless they find some means of expression, they are unknown and, for all practical purposes, nonexistent . . . what we might have been will never be known and is, therefore, not a part of the self. These undeveloped potentialities may be kept out of awareness because of the fear of anxiety, but this would be true only if there had been some attempt to express them which was frustrated by disapproval . . .
>
> Nevertheless, most of us, at least in the Western culture, treasure the notion of having an unique individual self. It is certainly a wide-spread belief, and one which is incidentally encouraged in our society. . . . As I have said it is a socially acceptable idea. Individualistic cultures at any rate encourage it interpersonal theory has no place for such a concept, except as an illusion encouraged by an individualistic culture. However, I do not see that interpersonal theory either affirms or denies its existence. Those who wish to believe it are just as free to do so as those who wish to deny it. It is beyond any scientific proof available to us at present. What interpersonal theory does establish is that even if we are entirely the products of interpersonal experience, each one is unique because his experience with other people is unique and the potentialities of his protoplasm are unique . . . each one of us has his own interpersonal experience which makes him different from everyone else.

(pp. 15–17)

Anna Antonovsky (1987)[13] opined that Thompson was "more inclined to allow for normative developmental ideas and for a potential and flexibility of the self beyond the strictly empirical limits that Sullivan had indicated."

(p. 548)

Thompson made use of some of Sullivan's techniques in her own work. Just as she made use of her collaborative work with Sándor Ferenczi.

The influence of Ferenczi's concept of the "dialogue of unconscious" can be heard in Thompson's conception of direct psychoanalytic experience. She acknowledges how two people can come to comprehend each other without any conscious experience of that nonverbal understanding (Ferenczi, 1915). That phenomenon of unconscious communication has come to be seen as an essential aspect of the psychoanalytic process and praxis.

Likewise, Ferenczi's theory of human growth focused on a type of unconditional "maternal" love that Thompson reformulated and expanded, contrasting the "need" for love with the "demand" for love.

> I think Ferenczi was not entirely clear on this matter. His idea was that the analyst must give the patient all the love he needs. The basic need of every child is to be accepted, to feel himself secure with one individual. This type of acceptance is also what the patient needs. I think, however, Ferenczi tended to confuse the idea that the patient must be given all the love he needs with the idea he must be given all the love he demands. Obviously, the two are not identical.
>
> (1943b, p. 64)

Thompson's work integrates an American understanding of psychoanalytic concepts with American feminism and a democratic sense of equality. This is an example of how her work remains relevant and living, beyond her time.

Clara Thompson entered the field of psychoanalysis on the ground floor. She became one of its significant contributors, establishing an American psychoanalytic tradition that shifted from discovering the workings of the analysand's mind to uncovering the dynamic nature of the relationship between the patient and the analyst, the interpersonal psychoanalytic tradition. She added a cultural perspective that shaped the field in the decades that followed. With her colleagues in America, she brought aspects of psychoanalysis's past into the future, as they explored new elements of the analytic relationship.

She also contributed to a psychoanalytically informed psychology of women that is taken up in the next chapter.

Notes

1 These reviews include, but are not limited to, Jung's (1933) *Modern Man in Search of a Soul*; Pearson's (1936b) "Speech Defect (Word Mutilation) and Masochism in a Traumatic Neurosis"; Schilder's (1936a) "The Attitude of Psychoneurotics Towards Death"; Coleman's (1937b) "August Strindberg: The Autobiographies"; Schilder's (1937) "Remarks on the Psychophysiology of the Skin"; Engle's (1937e) "A Study of Castration"; Kanzer's (1937d) "Personality of the Scientist"; Horney's (1937) "The Problem of Feminine Masochism" and The Neurotic Personality of our Time.

2 He was also an activist who opened up poetry to writers of color and young writers through his friendship with June Jordan, the Jamaican-American, self-identified bi-sexual poet. Brand refused to testify at the McCarthy hearings against his fellow writers at the League of American Writers. Thompson's choice of Brand to represent her work reflects her values—and possibly her relationship with Brand.

3 Given Sullivan's insight into the needs of gay men on the unit at Phipps, perhaps he might have dealt differently with Marian's anxiety and defenses. While Thompson was in consultation with Ferenczi about the case, we can't know if she also discussed it with Sullivan. Did she consult Izette de Forest who was having an affair with Alice Lowell? So much is unknown.

4 Up until the introduction of the journal, the premiere psychoanalytic journal was *International Journal of Psychoanalysis*.

5 Also in the issue is Lucile Dooley's "The Genesis of Psychological Sex Differences" (1938). Dooley often reappears in Thompson's life story. She was responsible for getting Thompson her first job and remained her friend throughout life, despite Dooley having held onto Freudian biological determinism (Peters, 1979). Her writing on the genesis of psychological sex differences is orthodox in this theoretical position. Other articles in *Psychiatry* carry an interdisciplinary imprint, including Thompson's essay—which reflects the influence of Ferenczi and is perhaps a nod to his request for her to bring back his ideas to America.

6 Fromm wrote: "Sigmund Freud had the tragic fate of seeing some of his most gifted pupils (Adler, Jung and Rank) leave him and become leaders of rival schools. . . . Only one of Freud's early collaborators did not leave the master, though he criticized and deviated essentially he was Sándor Ferenczi."

7 Adrienne Rich (1977) recalls her "black mother," in the context of African American mothering in segregated Baltimore in the 1930s around the same time Thompson and Fisher met.

> We are, none of us, either mother or daughters; to our amazement, confusion, and greater complexity, we are both. Women, mothers or not, who feel committed to other women, are increasingly giving each other a quality of caring filled with the diffuse kinds of identifications that exist between actual mothers and daughters.
>
> (p. 253)

8 Belkin (2021) points out,

> Because psychoanalysis focuses on both collective and individual trauma, it is uniquely positioned to address the effects of prejudice and discrimination. In our psychoanalytic work with marginalized patients, we need to explore their struggles through the combined lens of race, gender, and sexuality. We must keep in mind that homophobia, racism, and misogyny often operate in tandem, rather than separately.
>
> (p. 206)

9 Rich (1977), speaking to a time when she left her parent's house, recalls her "black mother" saying, "Yes, I understand how you have to leave and do what you think is right. I once had to break somebody's heart to go and live my life" (p. 254).

10 Sullivan noted: The Tragedy of the Negro in America seems to be chiefly a matter of culturally determined attitudes in the whites. . . . However, when the techniques of intensive study of interpersonal relations have been substituted for those of a detached and generally preoccupied professional man, the presumptively "typical Negro" performances have been resolved into particular instances of the typically human (Wake, 2011, p. 110).

11 Wake (2011) provides the example of the anthropologist Ruth Benedict, a friend of Thompson, who was entangled in a public/private dissonance. On the one hand, Benedict focused on the "bias against homosexuality as socially constructed bigotry" (p. 130), arguing that the stigmatization of homosexuality must be changed:

> A tendency toward [homosexuality] in our culture exposes an individual to all the conflicts . . . and we tend to identify the consequences of this conflict with homosexuality. But these consequences are obviously local and cultural. . . . Whenever homosexuality has been given an honorable place in any society, those to whom it is congenial have filled adequately the honorable roles.
>
> (Benedict, 1934, p. 64)

However, privately Ruth Benedict kept her relationship with Margaret Mead an open secret, much the way that Harry Stack Sullivan kept his relationship with James Inscoe secret to avoid shame and disapproval or worse. And yet, Sullivan's letters are replete with loving references to James (see Blitsten letters held in the Ralph Crowley papers).

12 The draft of the talk is not dated but we can assume it was written following Sullivan's death in 1949. The essay was published in 1958.

13 Antonovsky also found that Thompson "seemed to accept Erich Fromm's view that Sullivan's concept of the self was itself an expression of the alienated social character dominant in our age. She said that Sullivan had limited his field of observation to man's attempt to fit into our specific society and that he did not concern himself with unrealized potential, with what man might become in other circumstances. Because of this limitation, she stated, Sullivan "has only vague things to say about maturity. . . . He has practically nothing to say about mature love. He does define what passes for love at the juvenile and preadolescent levels" (p. 548).

References

Antonovsky, A. M. (1987). Object relations theory and interpersonal theory: Some comparative comments. *Psychoanalysis and Contemporary Thought*, *10*(4), 533–555.

Belkin, M. (2021). Intersectionality and psychoanalysis. *Contemporary Psychoanalysis*, *57*, 163–164.

Benedict, R. (1934). Anthropology and the abnormal. *The Journal of General Psychology*, *10*(1), 59–82.

Benedict, R. (1938). Continuities and discontinuities in cultural conditioning. *Psychiatry*, *1*(2), 161–167.

Brennan, B. W. (2009). Ferenczi's forgotten messenger: The life and work of Izette de Forest. *American Imago*, *66*(4), 427–455.

Carlyle, T. (1841). *On Heros, hero worship and the heroic in history*. New York: Adams.

de Forest, I. (1942). The therapeutic technique of Sándor Ferenczi. *International Journal of Psychoanalysis*, *23*, 120–139.

de Forest, I. (1954). *The leaven of love: A development of the psychoanalytic theory and technique of Sándor Ferenczi*. New York: Harper & Bros.

D'Ercole, A. (2017). The repossession of the interpersonal tradition: On holding close our transdisciplinary roots. *Contemporary Psychoanalysis*, *53*(1), 95–111.

Dooley, L. (1938). The genesis of psychological sex differences. *Psychiatry*, *1*(2), 181–195.

Ferenczi, S. (1915). Psychogenic anomalies of voice production. In S. Ferenczi (Ed.), *Further contributions to the theory and technique of psychoanalysis* (pp. 105–109). London: Karnac Books.

Ferenczi, S. (1928). The elasticity of the psychoanalytic technique. In S. Ferenczi (Ed.), *Final contributions to the problems and methods of psychoanalysis* (pp. 87–101). London: Karnac Books.

Frazier, E. F. (1939). *The Negro family in the United States*. Chicago: University of Chicago Press.

Frie, R., & Sauvayre, P. (2022). *Breaking boundaries: The interdisciplinary foundation of interpersonal psychoanalysis*. Routledge Press.

Fromm, E. (1955, August 7). Love stood between him and Freud. Review of the book, *The leaven of love* by I. de Forest. *New York Times*.

Fromm, E. (1956, March 11). *Thompson letter to Fromm*. Tubingen: Erich Fromm Archives.

Fromm, E. (1968, April 5). Letter to Ralph Crawley. The Oskar Diethelm Library, DeWitt Wallace Institute for the History of Psychiatry. The Weill Cornell Medical College, The Ralph Crowley Papers, Box 5, Fol. 7., New York, NY.

Gabbard, G. O. (2016). *Boundaries and boundary violations in psychoanalysis*. Washington, DC: American Psychiatric Publishing.

Green, M. R. (Ed.). (1964a). *Interpersonal psychoanalysis: The selected papers of Clara M. Thompson*. New York: Basic Books.

Green, M. R. (1964b). Her life. In M. R. Green (Ed.), *Interpersonal psychoanalysis: The selected papers of Clara M. Thompson.* pp. 347–377 New York: Basic Books.

Haas, A. P., & Drescher, J. (2014). Impact of sexual orientation and gender identity on suicide risk: Implications for assessment and treatment. *Psychiatric Times, 30*(12), 24–25.

Hanfmann, E. & Kasanin, J. (1942). Psychoanalysis and conditioned reflex. In E. Hanfmann & J. Kasanin (Eds.), *Conceptual thinking in Schizophrenia. Nervous and mental disease monographs.* New york, 1942.

Kamiat, P. (1939). *Social forces in personality stunting.* Cambridge, MA: Sci-Art Publishers.

Kay, J. (2014). Commentary on Clara Thompson's transference as a therapeutic instrument: Foreseeing the real relationship. *Psychiatry, Spring, 77*(1), 1–7.

McElya, M. (2007). *Clinging to mammy: The faithful slave in twentieth-century America.* Cambridge, MA: Harvard University Press.

Perry, H. S. (1982). *Psychiatrist of America: The life of Harry Stack Sullivan.* Cambridge, MA: Belknap Press.

Peters, M. (1979). Biographies of women. *Biography, 2*(3), 201–217.

Rachman, A. W. (1997). *Sándor Ferenczi: The psychotherapist of tenderness and passion.* New York: Jason Arson.

Rich, A. (1977). *Of woman born: Motherhood as experience and institution.* New York: W. W. Norton.

Shindler, P. (1936). Remarks on the psychophysiology of the skin. *Psychoanalytic Review, 23*(3), 274–285.

Silverberg, W. V. (1959). Clara Thompson memorial. *The Newsletter of the White Institute, 7*(1).

Sullivan, H. S. (1938). Introduction to the study of interpersonal relations. *Psychiatry, 1*(1).

Thompson, C. (1930). Analytic observations during the course of a manic-depressive psychosis. *Psychoanalytic Review, 17*(2), 240–252.

Thompson, C. (1931). " 'Dutiful child' resistance. *Psychoanalytic Review, 18*(4), 426–433.

Thompson, C. (1934) *Modern Man in Search of a Soul:* By C. G. Jung. (Harcourt, Brace & Co., New York, 1933. pp. 282). *International Journal of Psychoanalysis, 15,* 349–350.

Thompson, C. (1936) Children: Gerald H. J. Pearson. 'Speech Defect (Word Mutilation) and Masochism in a Traumatic Neurosis.' *Psycho-analytic Review,* January 1936, Vol. XXIII, pp. 46–58. *International Journal of Psychoanalysis, 17,* 232.

Thompson, C. (1936). Clinical: Paul Schilder. 'Remarks on the Psychophysiology of the Skin.' *Psychoanalytic Review,* 1936, *23*(3), pp. 274–285.

Thompson, C. (1937) Applied: Stanley M. Coleman. 'August Strindberg: the Autobiographies.' *Psychoanalytic Review,* 1936, *23*(3) pp. 248–273. *International Journal of Psychoanalysis, 18,* 313–314.

Thompson, C. (1937) Clinical: Paul Schilder. 'Remarks on the Psychophysiology of the Skin.' *Psychoanalytic Review*, 1936, *23*(3), pp. 274–285. *International Journal of Psychoanalysis*, *18*, 63.

Thompson, C. (1937) General: Bernice S. Engle, A.M. 'Attis.—A Study of Castration.' *Psychoanalytic Review*, 1936, Vol. 23, pp. 363–372. *International Journal of Psychoanalysis*, *18*, 58.

Thompson, C. (1937) General: Mark G. Kanzer. 'Personality of the Scientist.' *Psychoanalytic Review*, 1936, Vol. 23, pp. 373–382. *International Journal of Psychoanalysis*, *18*, 57–58.

Thompson, C. (1937) Sexuality: Karen Horney. 'The Problem of Feminine Masochism.' *Psycho-analytic Review*, July, 1935, *23*(3), pp. 241–257. *International Journal of Psychoanalysis*, *18*, 64–65.

Thompson, C. (1937) The Neurotic Personality of our Time: By Karen Horney. (New York, W. W. Norton & Co. pp. 290 and Index. $3.00.). *International Journal of Psychoanalysis*, *18*, 315–316.

Thompson, C. (1938b). Development of awareness of transference in a markedly detached personality. *International Journal of Psychoanalysis*, *19*, 299–309.

Thompson, C. (1938c). Notes on the psychoanalytic significance of the choice of analyst. *Psychiatry*, *1*(2), 205–216.

Thompson, C. (1939). Review of the book *Thalassa: A theory of genitality* by S. Ferenczi. *Psychiatry*, *2*, 138.

Thompson, C. (1940a). Review of the book *Social forces in personality stunting* by A. H. Kamiat. *Psychoanalytic Quarterly*, *9*, 572–572.

Thompson, C. (1940b). Identification with the enemy and loss of the sense of self. *Psychoanalytic Quarterly*, *9*(1), 37–50.

Thompson, C. (1941). The role of women in this culture. *Psychiatry*, *4*(1), 1–8.

Thompson, C. (1942). Cultural pressures in the psychology of women. *Psychiatry*, *5*(3), 331–339.

Thompson, C. (1943a). "Penis envy" in women. *Psychiatry*, *6*(2), 123–125.

Thompson, C. (1943b). "The therapeutic technique of Sándor Ferenczi": A comment. *International Journal of Psychoanalysis*, *24*, 64–66.

Thompson, C. (1945). Transference as a therapeutic instrument. *Psychiatry*, *8*(3), 273–278.

Thompson, C. (1946). Review of the book *Conceptual thinking in schizophrenia* by E. Hanfmann and J. S. Kasanin. *Psychoanalytic Review*, *33*(3), 383–384.

Thompson, C. (1947). Changing concepts of homosexuality in psychoanalysis. *Psychiatry*, *X*, 183–189.

Thompson, C. (1949). Cultural conflicts of women in our society. *Samiksa*, *3*, 125–134.

Thompson, C. (1950a). *Psychoanalysis: Evolution and development*. New York: Hermitage.

Thompson, C. (1950b). Some effects of the derogatory attitude towards female sexuality. *Psychiatry*, *13*(3), 349–354.

Thompson, C. (1952). Countertransference. *Samiksa*, *4*(4), 205–211.

Thompson, C. (1953). Transference and character analysis. *Samiksa, 7,* 260–270.

Thompson, C. (1956). The role of the analyst's personality in therapy. *American Journal of Psychotherapy, 10*(2), 347–367.

Thompson, C. (1958a). Concepts of the self in interpersonal theory. *American Journal of Psychotherapy, 12*(1), 5–17.

Thompson, C. (1958b). A study of the emotional climate of psychoanalytic institutes. *Psychiatry, 21*(1), 45–51.

Thompson, C. (1959a). Dynamics of hostility: A panel discussion (with F. A. Weiss, B. Zuger, C. Thompson, L. Landman, & J. A. Meerloo). *American Journal of Psychoanalysis, 19*(1), 10–13.

Thompson, C. (1959b). Un estudio del clima emocional de los institutos psicoanalíticos. *Revista de psicoanálisis, 16*(1), 49–57.

Thompson, C. (1959c). An introduction to minor maladjustments. In S. Arieti (Ed.), *American handbook of psychiatry* (pp. 237–244). New York: Basic Books.

Thompson, C. (1978). Sullivan and psychoanalysis. *Contemporary Psychoanalysis, 14*(4), 488–501.

Thompson, C. (1979). Sullivan and Fromm. *Contemporary Psychoanalysis, 15*(2), 195–200.

Thompson, C. (1988). Sándor Ferenczi, 1873–1933. *Contemporary Psychoanalysis, 24*(2), 182–195.

Thompson, C. (2017). The history of the William Alanson White Institute. *Contemporary Psychoanalysis, 53*(1), 7–28.

Wake, N. (2011). *Private practices: Harry Stack Sullivan, the science of homosexuality, and American liberalism.* New Brunswick, NJ: Rutgers University Press.

Wallace-Sanders, K. (2008). *Mammy: A century of race, gender and southern memory.* MI: University of Michigan. Ann Arbor.

Waugaman, R. M. (2016). Further notes on choosing an analyst. *Psychiatry, 79*(1), 13–18.

William Alanson White Institute. (1938). Unindexed from matter. *Psychiatry, 1*(1), i–vii.

Chapter 5

Evolution Revolution

Thompson's Psychology of Women

How did Clara Thompson move from her conservative religious training to her pioneering ideas about women and society? Certainly, the injunction from her teachers at Pembroke not to 'take ideas off the counter' but to think critically helped her make fundamental choices about the world despite the accompanying anxiety. She made bold choices for a woman in the early days of the 20th century, even for a privileged American white woman.

Years before Clara Thompson was born, the 1848 Seneca Falls Convention called on all American women to fight for women's constitutional right to equality, which included the right to vote, hold property, and obtain an education. Thompson's hometown of Rhode Island had its own Women's Suffrage Association that actively fought for the rights of women; these sentiments were in the air and no doubt influenced Thompson's budding feminism. Her connections with the leaders of the culture-and-personality school[1] also infused her theories on the psychology of women.

In her scholarship, Thompson turned toward the past to comprehend the present while looking to science—in findings from anthropologists and sociologists. As Capelle (1998) explains,

> Mead and Benedict's colleague Edward Sapir (1932) wrote that "cultural anthropology . . . has the healthiest of all skepticism's about the validity of the concept 'normal behavior'" (p. 235). In the 1940s and 1950s, Thompson was the only "cultural school" analyst to apply this skepticism to the question of woman's nature and carry culturalist premises to their logical conclusions. She was alone in her insistence that what seemed to be inherent femininity was most likely the result of cultural conditioning. Sullivan was not willing to go that far, and neither was Fromm."

> (p. 88)

DOI: 10.4324/9781003284840-6

Thompson presented her paper, "What Is Penis Envy?" on May 19, 1941, at the first annual convention of the Association for The Advancement of Psychoanalysis held in conjunction with the American Psychiatric Association. This was the first year of the new organization following the walkout from New York Psychoanalytic. The morning sessions were dedicated to a panel on human destructiveness.[2] In the afternoon, Clara Thompson took to the podium to present her paper. She explains the origins of the term, "penis envy,"

> [It's] a term coined by Freud and used by him to describe a basic attitude found in neurotic women. The term had more than symbolic meaning to him. He was convinced that this envy in women grew out of a feeling of biological lack beginning with the little girl's discovery in early childhood that she lacked something possessed by the little boy. Because of this, according to Freud, she believed she had been castrated, and she dealt with this shock either by sublimating the wish for a penis in the wish for a child; i.e., becoming a normal woman, or by the development of neurosis, or by a character change described as the masculinity complex, a type of character which seeks to deny that any lack exists.
>
> (p. 1)[3]

She disagreed with Freud's phallocentric views. She felt that Freud held too much power over psychoanalysts' perspectives on women's psychology.

Fueled in part by the work of Karen Horney who she credits, Thompson's views held firmly to cultural considerations more than her predecessors.[4] She challenged psychoanalysts to think of equality—fairness, equal opportunity, sameness—not gender difference. Her cultural analysis was generative of future psychoanalytic feminism, but it took years for that to take hold.

She viewed biological differences as differences that did not warrant either discrimination or distinctiveness as she argued that these differences were not reasons to find women significantly less or more than men. Biology, specifically, "the lack of a penis," she argued, "did not shape one's personality or internal life" as Freud maintained. Thompson consistently relied on social inequalities as explanations for gendered behavior.

Capelle (1998) submits that her ideas about culture may have "offered a means of understanding her experience and validating her chosen path, her interests and ambitions" (1998, p. 90). Thompson stood outside of the feminist psychoanalytic circle with her cultural analysis of women's psychology as she challenged Freud's view of women as she argued that a patriarchal culture imposed limits on women, not their biology. The more popular thread of discourse in feminist theorizing in the 1940s was grounded in the matriarchal religious premises of Johann Jakob Bachofen's (see *Myth, Religion, and Mother Right*, 1992).[5] Bachofen posited a prehistoric matriarchy where social life was hypothesized within a mother–child bond connected to nature and instincts. As a mystic, Bachofen was interested in the inner life of human beings. Among those influenced by Bachofen were Georg Groddeck,[6] Karen Horney, and Erich Fromm (Friedman, 2013). Bachofen's view of a matriarchal era elevated women's powerlessness to powerfulness by virtue of their biology. Within that framework, women's biological differences from men, for example, menstruation, pregnancy, childbirth, and breastfeeding bestowed special characterological qualities. Unlike Horney and Fromm, Thompson was not influenced by Bachofen's or Freud's way of thinking. She was drawn to the theories of anthropologists and sociologists that addressed social conditioning.

In March of 1950,[7] Thompson presented the paper again at a symposium, "Feminine Psychology: Its Implications for Psychoanalytic Medicine."[8] By now she had broken with Karen Horney and had established the William Alanson White Institute. Summarizing Elizabeth Capelle's (1993) reporting, one of the organizers of the day's events thought it would be a "Feast of love" that would bring together various psychoanalytic factions with shared clinical interests (Capelle, p. 379). Thompson challenged Freudian theory in her retitled paper, "On Cultural Complications in the Sexual Life of Women" with the subtitle, "Some Effects of the Deprecatory Attitude Towards Female Sexuality" (1950) and presented it to a packed crowd in the auditorium. Capelle makes the point that her colleagues did not support her position. Was it because she was critical of Freud's theory of female sexuality, or because she dared to be critical of her male mentors, Ferenczi and Fromm? Thompson felt that men spoke on the topic of female sexuality with no experience of the issues. Or because she accused her analytic peers, like the "unnamed Helene Deutsch" of being dominated by Freud's thinking (Capelle, 1993, p. 380). She thought they minimized the sexual needs of women and saw men's sexual drives as paramount. She found Fromm's thesis in "Sex and Character" (1943) particularly troublesome.[9] He had argued that

the ability to perform is important in male sexual life, that it is especially a matter of concern to the male because it is not entirely within his control, and that the female may perform at all times if she so wishes.

(Thompson, 1950a, p. 349)

She also disagreed with Ferenczi on the topic because he theorized that identification with the male in his orgasm constitutes a woman's true sexual fulfillment (pp. 349–354).

Thompson explained that she and Horney had previously published critical evaluations of Freud's theory on the topic of penis envy in *New Ways in Psychoanalysis* (1939) and in her essays "The Role of Women in this Culture" (1941) and "Cultural Pressures in the Psychology of Women" (1942). In "Penis Envy" in Women, Thompson points to how "cultural factors can explain the tendency of women to feel inferior about their sex and their consequent tendency to envy men" (1943, p. 123).

This situation, she argues, "can lead women to blame all their difficulties on their sex" (p. 123).

> Thus one can say the term "penis envy" is a symbolic representation of the attitude of women in this culture, a picturesque way of referring to the types of warfare which so often goes on between men and women. . . . It seems clear that envy of the male exists in most women in this culture, that there is a warfare between the sexes. The question to be considered is whether this warfare is different in kind from other types of struggle which go on between humans and if it is not actually different, why is there such preoccupation with the difference in sex?
>
> I believe that the manifest hostility between men and women is not different in kind from any other struggle between combatants, one of whom has definite advantage in prestige and position.
>
> (pp. 123–124)

Obvious Differences

Thompson explains why we use body parts to explain our differences.

> Two things have contributed to giving the fact of sexual difference a false importance.' Penis envy and castration ideas are common in dreams, symptoms and other manifestations of unconscious thinking. Body parts and functions are frequent symbols in archaic thought.

These ideas then may be only the presentation of other problems in symbolic body terms. There is not necessarily any evidence that the body situation is the cause of the thing it symbolizes. Any threat to the personality may appear in a dream as a castration. Furthermore, there is always a temptation to use some obvious situation as a rationalization of a more obscure one.

(p. 124)

Her pragmatic appraisals are compelling. She explains,

Sexual difference is an obvious difference, and obvious differences are especially convenient marks of derogation in any competitive situation in which one group aims to get power over the other.

She continues to argue that both feelings of inferiority as well as justifications for superiority are often made based on "easily recognizable" differences and provides the comparison of skin color. She argues,
    "Discrimination because of color is a case in point. Here, a usually easily distinguishable difference is a sign which taken as adequate justification for gross discrimination and underprivilege."

(p. 124)

She adds,

Few indeed of the governing class can be so fatuous as to believe that black skin implies an intrinsic inferiority. It is amazing, however, to discover how near to this superficiality many of their rationalizations actually come.

(p. 124)

She returns to sexual difference and underscores again,

The penis or lack of penis is another easily distinguishable mark of difference and is used in a similar manner. That is, the penis is the sign of the person in power in one particular competitive setup in this culture, that between man and woman. The attitude of the women in this situation is not qualitatively different from that found in any minority group in a competitive culture. So, the attitude called penis envy is similar to the attitude of any underprivileged group toward those in power.

(p. 124)

How progressive for Thompson to write about racial inequality in the context of gender inequality. She understood the role of power in the fight for sexual and for racial equity. Her comments are straightforward and bold.

She also contends that sexual difference has a "false importance" (p. 124).

> Penis envy and castration are frequent in dreams and other manifestations of unconscious thinking. Body parts and functions are frequent symbols in archaic thought. These ideas may be only the presentation of other problems in symbolic body terms. There is not necessarily any evidence that the body situation is the cause of the thing it symbolizes. Any threat to the personality may appear in a dream as a castration . . . there is always a temptation to use some obvious situation as a rationalization of a more obscure one. The penis envy concept offers women an explanation for their feelings of inadequacy by referring it to an evidently irremediable cause. In the same way, it offers the man a justification for his aggression against her.
>
> (p. 124)

She also speaks to how envy is a characteristic of a competitive culture and gives three examples.

> One does away with envy by achieving success. If one fails in proving that one is as good or better than the envied one, tendencies to revenge may develop. The person seeks then to pull the superior one down and in some way humiliate him. Or a person may withdraw from competition, apparently have no ambition, and desire to be inconspicuous. In such a situation, although there may be a feeling of helplessness and increased dependency, there may also be a secret feeling of power from being aloof to the struggle.
>
> (pp. 124–125)

While Thompson was writing in the 1940s, the enduringness of the concept of penis envy in psychoanalysis was still questioned three decades later, when the psychoanalyst Elsa First (1974), reviewing *Psychoanalysis and Feminism* by Juliet Mitchell (1947), provocatively asks,

> Ah, penis envy! Is it on its way to becoming a topic for nostalgia, taking its place in the museum along with chastity belts and corsets?
>
> (p. 382)

Thompson argued that the meaning of the anatomical difference between the sexes relies on a patriarchal culture; she would not sign on to the notion that culture shaped the psyche in quite the way that Juliet Mitchell proposed.[10] Rather Thompson's analysis of gender evolved from her own childhood experiences where gender roles were fixed within a theocratic system that encouraged boys to participate in the world and girls to take care of the needs of others, which included spiritual needs through missionary work. Once she discarded that bias, she was free to think and speak her feminist mind within the constraints of the era in which she lived.

Thompson was decidedly feminist in her discussion of envy.

> In patriarchal culture the restricted opportunities afforded women, the limitations placed on her development and independence give a real basis for envy of the male quite apart from any neurotic trends . . . the traditional family is no longer of central importance, the specific biological female contribution, the bearing of children, loses value coordinate with the various factors which encourage a diminishing birth rate. This although it is not a biologic inferiority, acts as if it were in that a woman can feel that what she has specifically to contribute is not needed or desired.
>
> Therefore, two situations in the culture are of importance in this discussion: the general tendency to be competitive which stimulates envy; and the tendency to place an inferior evaluation on women.
>
> (p. 125)

On Not Touching the Future

The suffragists (often referred to as the first wave of the woman's movements) argued for sexual [gender] equality, as did the radical wing of the Free Will Baptist Women's Missionary group who in ways echoed that feminist effort. The spirit of feminism guided Thompson into adulthood. It comes as no surprise that she would see the problems women face as issues of social inequality. Her perspective was binary, historical, cultural, and liberal, confirming the idea that the government should "do something" following the findings of science to solve perceived social problems.

She urged psychoanalysts to contemplate both the social and psychological worlds of their patients and to consider the conditions in American culture that produce and sustain gender inequity.

Through a Feminist Lens

The second-wave feminism's axiom "the personal is political"—a feminist cry to action, brought the discussion of women's subjective experiences into the political arena, it was ahead of Thompson's theorizing. The personal is political-infused women's stories by hearing individual experiences as part of the political situation of women's inequality. Thompson did incorporate her patients' experiences to build her theory. Her approach opened a path for women in the future to contemplate the effects of the pernicious and insistent sexism that haunted their lives. It is important to hold in mind that she is writing these texts in the mid-1940s through the 1950s, following the Second World War. It was a time of stultifying conservativism that sent women back into domesticity. It was also a time of binary thinking about gender.[11]

The psychoanalyst, Sue Shapiro (2002) grounded in her knowledge of both psychoanalytic history and academic feminist scholarship provides an important and personal account of the history of feminism and interpersonal psychoanalysis. She points to how "feminism as a political movement "changed the lives of women and their opportunities for education, work, a political voice, sexual pleasure, financial independence, power, and authority" (p. 215). Her narrative begins when she was a graduate student seeking to situate herself within the world of women psychoanalysts. As she searched for a role model among the women who populated the field, she questioned where she would fit. She wrote the essay in memory of Ruth Moulton and in recognition of early women in the field. She concludes, "I needed to find my way to a woman who, like Clara Thompson, recognized the need for creating and accepting alternative life choices for women—choices that could include single parenting, serial monogamy, or even some form of communal living (p. 248). Thompson was a role model for many women.

There are many excellent accounts of psychoanalysis and feminism (see Capelle, 1998; Chodorow, 1978; Mitchell, 1974; Gallop, 1982; Benjamin, 1988; Dimen (1995), to name a few) that examine the historical interface and questions concerning our psychic lives and social existence. I circle back to the historical analysis provided in Elizabeth Capelle's (1993) dissertation, *Analyzing the "modern woman": Psychoanalytic Debates about feminism, 1920–1950* and to her essay *Clara Thompson as a Culturalist* (1998). Capelle's analysis is a vital source of information about Thompson, particularly as an intellectual history of early psychoanalytic debates about feminism. I have drawn liberally from her work. Her elaboration of the "continental view" and the "Anglo-American view" offers a way of distinguishing these positions in late 19th- and early 20th-century feminism. She explains,

> to a much greater extent than their Anglo-American contemporaries, continental feminists assumed that women were equal to men, but different from them, and that the essence of woman's difference lay in her maternalism.
>
> (Capelle, 1993, p. 9)

Maternal capacities became a persistent and controversial focal point in the discussion of women's psychology. Chodorow (1978), who turned to the cultural school of psychoanalysts, cites Erich Fromm, Karen Horney, and Clara Thompson as those who were critical of Freud's instinct theory of development. Chodorow's thesis that "women's mothering perpetuates itself through social-structurally induced psychological mechanisms" would have appealed to Thompson but the emphasis on mothering may have turned her away (Chodorow, 1978, p. 211).

Sue Shapiro (2002) clarifies,

> In both political and theoretical feminism there is an ongoing debate between the "difference feminists," who valorize women and their experience, which they view as essentially different from men's experience, and the "egalitarian/gender critique feminists," who challenge essentialist thinking about both men and women. This division of feminists was originally noted by Dimen (1995), who coined the term "gender critique feminists" in the course of laying out the debate.
>
> (p. 217)

Dimen (1995) in her discussion of "gender critique feminists" speaks to how Freud used "what anthropologists call 'folk science,' . . . to codify unexamined popular assumptions about women and, implicitly men." She notes that in the last of his essays on femininity Freud firmed up his view concluding:

> Women were castrated, penisless men who suffered from penis envy and morally inferior weak superegos. They could achieve femininity only by abandoning their clitoral, deemed "masculine," sexuality in

favor of the vaginal orgasm. Their only hope for feminine fulfillment was through mothering and the acquisition of the baby that would serve them as a symbolic penis.

(p. 304)

Dimen identifies how Thompson located penis envy not in a body part but in women's standing in society.

{Freud's} "depreciation of a specifically feminine sexuality and his ignorance of the powers and joys of motherhood derived from prevailing cultural misogyny. . . . Thompson, in turn, located *women's* envy in society. . . . She argued that women's feelings of inferiority and injury, or what Freud would have called penis envy, emerge from their lesser social and economic standing."

(p. 304)

For Thompson it was always culture that presented women with conflicts between work and love—conflicts she argued, men did not have to face.

During the 1940s, Thompson moved further into the culturalist position. Consistent with her early educational emphasis, she stressed that society changes to meet individuals' needs for self-realization. In her {Thompson's} 1937 review of Karen Horney's essay "The Problem of Feminine Masochism" she notes:

The paper begins by raising two questions (1) How far is masochism of the essence of the female? and (2) How far have social conditionings influenced the formation of her masochistic trends? The tentative conclusion of the paper is that social conditioning is probably the more important factor of the two. . . . The biological sexual functions have in themselves no masochistic connotations, but certain things may be given a masochistic meaning when masochistic needs of other origin are present. Such meaning may be given (1) the greater average physical strength of men, (2) the possibility of rape, (3) the pain of menstruation, defloration and child-birth, and (4) the being penetrated in intercourse. These give a woman a certain preparedness for a masochistic conception of her role. This preparedness without the conditioning of the culture probably does not develop as judged by the disappearance of masochistic trends through analysis.

(pp. 64–65)

Thompson credits Horney's (1937) *The Neurotic Personality of Our Time* as,

> one of the first definite presentations of a new orientation stressing
> the importance of cultural and environmental influences in neurosis.
> It has been said that Freud always took cultural forces into considera-
> tion, and it is probable that he did so even more than he himself knew.
> However, his theoretical approach stressed biology. The new approach
> discarded the libido theory and presented a new concept of man and
> his relation to society.
>
> (p. 16)

Trained by first-generation interpersonal psychoanalysts, Ruth Moulton
(1975), analyzed by Clara Thompson, and supervised by Harry Stack Sullivan, Erich Fromm, and Frieda Fromm-Reichmann, evaluated the feminist
contributions of Karen Horney between 1922 and 1932 and Clara Thompson in the 1940s. Moulton[12] argues that Horney was "freer of a strong personal bond" to Freud than women who had worked closely with him such
as Helene Deutsch, Jeanne Lampl De Groot, Ruth Mack Brunswick, and
Marie Bonaparte (p. 210). Horney, she argued, made her "divergences with
Freud much clearer although she continued to use Freudian terms until
she came to America in 1932" (p. 210). Thompson had no direct connection with Freud and so could break more easily from Freudian theories.
But unlike Horney, she did not receive as much credit for her revisions.
Moulton suggests the reason for this is that Thompson's papers had a
"very pragmatic tone, sticking close to clinical observations of women in
their cultural milieu, with no effort to formulate new theories about them"
(p. 219). Along those lines, Capelle (1998) suggests Thompson offered a
"no fault feminism" or more critically, "feminism without politics" (p. 93).

My view is that Thompson's politics were decidedly feminist. Her clinical
attitudes underscored that social and political forces shape behavior. She blamed
discrimination and inequality solidly on culture and cultural conditioning.

> Women . . . have had difficult in freeing themselves from an idea
> which was a part of their life training. Thus it has come about that
> even when a women has become consciously convinced of the value
> she still has to contend with the unconscious effects of training, dis-
> crimination again her, and traumatic experiences which keep alive the
> attitude of inferiority.
>
> (Green, 1964, p. 233)

She saw a different patient population from Freud's and noted that women in America "are probably freer to live their own lives than in any other patriarchal country in the world. This does not mean to say that they have ceased to be an underprivileged group" (Thompson, 1941, p. 1). She drew from Fromm saying, "When a positive gain of a culture begins to fail, then restlessness comes until a new satisfaction is found" (p. 2).

Thompson's Psychology of Women

Thompson's first essay on women, "Female Adolescence," was written anonymously,[13] included in Sullivan's *Personal Psychopathology* (1965). The chapter gave her a forum for her thoughts on the topic. Sullivan may have changed some of the wording and the end of the chapter discusses the less-than-hopeful possibilities for women who want to enter what were considered male professions, medicine, law, etc. Sullivan was not particularly helpful on women's issues, but Fromm offered some practical analytic tools for her analysis of the aims of the modern woman. His theories on social character helped inform her work despite her disagreement with his views on women's sexuality. It was not unlike her to parse between ideas that made sense and those that did not.

Thompson's Four Essays on the Psychology of Women

In a set of four landmark essays published between 1941 and 1950, Thompson laid out her views on the psychology of women. In—"The Role of Women in This Culture" (1941); "Cultural Pressures in the Psychology of Women" (1942); " 'Penis Envy' in Women" (1943); and "Some Effects of the Derogatory Attitude toward Female Sexuality" (1950a); together with "Cultural Complications in the Sexual Life of Women" (1950b) and other of her essays that focused on women's biology and development across the lifespan (Green, 1964). She is pragmatic and straightforward, remaining close to her clinical observations as she offers a cultural analysis of the psychological problems women encounter in a patriarchal society.

In "The Role of Women in This Culture" (1941), she maintains she would make no attempt to study early conditioning and individual traumatic factors, because she was interested in demonstrating what women do to deal with their increased awareness of their cultural inferiority and how social pressure was causing psychological problems. This position is psychoanalytically interpersonal in its focus on what people do to cope with their situation, but it brought her criticism. Most forms of criticism viewed her as too sociological.

Thompson was a 20th-century feminist embedded in an era of social change that stopped short during the conservative era of the 1950s. Elucidating the progress from 1930 through the 1950s

Thompson begins as is typical qualifying what she aims to do:

> "The aim here is *merely* to present observations and speculations on the cultural problems seen through the eyes of psychoanalytic patients. This offers a limited but very important view of the situation."
>
> (p. 1, italics added)

She maintains "for economic reasons psychoanalysis is not yet available to any extent to the lower classes" (p. 1), she hopes that in the future a community psychoanalysis will be available. Sadly we are still awaiting a community psychoanalysis. Thompson points to how psychoanalysis is not everyone's interest, particularly individuals with "strong reactionary cultural attitudes" as well as, "individuals who are leading fairly contented lives" (p. 1). She reasons, American women are freer than women in most patriarchal countries but that does not mean they cease to be underprivileged. She points out there have always been,

> women who, by their cleverness or special circumstances, have been able to circumvent this position, but in general, the girl child has been trained from childhood to fit herself for her inferior role; and, as long as compensations were adequate, women have been relatively content . . . if in return for being a man's property a woman receives economic security, a full emotional life centering around husband and children, and an opportunity to express her capacities in the management of her home, she has little cause for discontent. The question of her inferiority scarcely troubles her when her life is happily fulfilled, even though she lives in relative slavery.
>
> Our problem with women today is not simply that they are caught in a patriarchal culture, but that they are living in a culture in which the positive gains for them are failing . . . on the other hand, the culture is beginning to offer her something positive in an opportunity to join in a life outside the home where she may compete with other women and even with men in business. In the sexual sphere, too, with the spread

of birth-control knowledge and a more open attitude in general about sex, there is an increasing tendency in and out of marriage to have a sexual life approximating in its freedom that enjoyed by the male. However, these things do not yet run smoothly . . . we are not yet dealing with a stable situation, but one in transition; therefore, one in which the individual is confused and filled with conflict, one in which old attitudes and training struggle with new ideas.

(p. 2)

Thompson was aware that the world was in transition. That she benefited from societal changes and that like other women she too was caught up in the pressures of social change.

Discrimination during the early 20th century was blatant.[14] At a minimum she endured what we refer to as "mansplaining" along with the condescending or patronizing behavior that comes with it. She noted how women had to,

work out a new way of life with no precedent to follow and no adequate training from early childhood to help them take the work drive seriously or fit it into their lives . . . when the individual has the courage in herself to attempt the new road, she has to cope with emotional pressures not only form society as a whole but from the individuals most important to her. One of the most significant of these pressures is the attitude of a prospective husband who has his own traditions and wishes for his future wife and, since he is often confused in his attempt to adjust to the new ways of life, may interpret the woman's struggle to find a place for herself as evidence of lack of love or a slur on his manhood.

(p. 3)

If she were writing from the future, she would have been able to tell "her story" with the emotional clarity we in the 21st century have grown accustomed. She did see that,

Social institutions put obstacles in the way of change of a woman's status. In the economic sphere she must usually accept a lower wage than men for the same type of work. She must be more capable than the man with whom she competes before she will be considered his equal.

(p. 4)

These observations were as relevant then as they are today. She suggests, "Even with increased economic freedom, there is considerable variation in the social satisfactions available to independent women" (p. 4).

Thompson sorts individuals into types as she discusses the problems they may encounter.

Some women who marry and have children may feel it is their duty and go about trying to prove their adequacy as a woman by having children.

> She may make a cult of her child, or she may play bridge or have some other play life, or she may engage in some volunteer employment. . . . Making a cult of the child is unfortunately a fairly frequent solution. By the term cult is here meant an anxious concern about the child's welfare where the mother goes to excessive lengths to apply all modern psychological and hygienic theories to the management of her child's development. This can be very destructive for the child. . . . Another type of woman finds in the marriage with no responsibility the fulfillment of her neurotic needs. This is the very infantile woman. For her marriage is a kind of sanitarium . . . those who work and do not marry, there are two main subdivisions. First . . . are those to whom work is everything; that is, there is no love life of significance . . . this group might be characterized as having found economic freedom without emotional freedom. . . . The second group are those who have a love life in addition to work. This love life may be homosexual or heterosexual, and the relationships may vary from the casual with frequent changes of partner to a fairly permanent relationship with one person, a relationship which may differ very little from marriage . . . there is one important difference from a married partnership. The individual considers herself free although she actually may be very involved emotionally. She regards her work as the most important and permanent thing in her life.
>
> (pp. 4–5)

This last characterization rings true for Thompson's life. No doubt she would have considered herself emotionally involved with Henry Major. They were not "free" to marry since Major was already married. If that were not a fact, would she have married him? What we can say is that for Thompson, her work was the most permanent part of her life.

She wraps up her comments asserting that,

> Inevitably, poorly adjusted people are in the vanguard of revolutionary movements. This one for the emancipation of women is certainly no exception. Women who studied medicine in the early years were on the whole those who had great personal problems about being women. Many a parallel example readily comes to mind. Some therapists may carry the marks of experience in those days. In any case, there is a temptation to view all change as neurotic. . . . Neurotic drives often find expression in the present-day activities of women but this is no reason for dismissing as neurotic the whole social and economic revolution of woman along her particular path among the worldwide changes.
>
> (p. 8)

In "Cultural Pressures in the Psychology of Women" (1942), Thompson examines the cultural influences leading to certain personality problems. She argues that a given culture tends to produce certain character types and trends.

> Most of these neurotic trends are found working similarly in both sexes. Thus, for example, the so-called masochistic character is by no means an exclusively feminine phenomenon. Likewise the neurotic need to be loved is often found dominating the life of men as well as women. The neurotic need of power and insatiable ambition drives are not only found in men, but also in women.
>
> Nevertheless, in some respects the problems of women are basically different from those of men. These fundamental differences are due to two things . . . woman has a different biologic function and because of this her position in society necessarily differs in some respects from that of the man. Second, the cultural attitude toward women differs significantly from that toward men for reason quite apart from biological necessity. These two differences present women with certain problems which men do not have to face.
>
> (p. 331)

She writes, "The official attitude of the culture toward women has been and still is to the effect that woman is not the equal of man" (p. 333), and then goes on to discuss how

> The culture invites masculinity in women. With the passing of the old sheltered life, with the increasing competition with men growing out of the industrial revolution as well as out of women's restlessness, it is not strange that her first steps toward equality would be in the direction of trying to be like men. Having no path of their own to follow women have tended to copy men. Imitating of a person superior to one is by no means unusual. The working man seeking to move up the social and economic scale not only tries to copy the middle-class way of life but may try to adopt the middle-class way of thinking. He may try so hard that he becomes a caricature of the thing he wishes to be, with loss of sight of his real goals in the process. In the same way, women, by aping men may develop a caricature situation and lose sight of their own interests. . . . It is true, practically speaking, that in the business and professional world it often paid to act like a man. Women were entering a domain which had been in the possession of men, in which the so-called masculine traits of decisiveness, daring, and aggression were usually far more effective than the customarily ascribed traits such as gentleness and submissiveness. In adaptation to this new way of life, woman could not but tend to change the personality traits acquired from their former cultural setting.
>
> (p. 338)

This is a very Frommian analysis. She writes,

> If a woman develops characteristics which indicate that she unconsciously considers herself a man, she is discontent with being a woman. It would be fruitful to inquire what this "being a woman" means to her. I have suggested the possibility of several unpleasant meanings. Being a woman may mean to her being inferior, being restricted, and being in the power of someone. In short, being a woman may mean negation of her feeling of self, a denial of the chance to be an independent person.
>
> (p. 339)

Wake (2011) reports that America's mass media held a "fascination with mannish women" and "effeminate men" (p. 2). She discusses how the most rampant government-led anti-homosexual campaigns were aimed at people who dared to even dress outside of traditional gender prescriptions to those who made a life and career outside traditional gender boundaries.

Thompson's "Some Effects of the Derogatory Attitude Toward Female Sexuality"[15] (1950a) picks up where she left off in her paper "Penis Envy" asserting:

> I stressed the fact that the actual envy of the penis as such is not as important in the psychology of women as their envy of the position of the male in our society. . . . That there are innate biological differences between the sexual life of man and woman is so obvious that one must apologize for mentioning it. Yet those who stress this aspect most are too often among the first to claim knowledge of the psychic experiences and feelings of the opposite sex. Thus, for many centuries male writers have been busy trying to attempt to explain the female. In recent years a few women have attempted to present the inner life of their own sex, but they themselves seem to have had difficulty in freeing their thinking from the male orientation. Psychoanalysts, female as well as male, seem for the most part still to be dominated by Freud's thinking about women.
>
> In the case of sexual experiences, however, one sex has no adequate means of identifying with the experience of the other sex. A woman, for instance, cannot possibly be sure that she knows what the subject is experience of an erection and male orgasm is. Nor can a man identify with the tension and sensations of menstruation, or female genital excitation, or childbirth. Since for many years most of the psychoanalysts were men this may account for the prevalence of some misconceptions about female sexuality.
>
> (p. 349)

Thompson objected to and questioned the views of two of her own mentors, Erich Fromm and Sándor Ferenczi. Ferenczi felt "inclined to think that identification with the male in his orgasm constitutes a woman's true sexual fulfillment" (p. 351). And, Fromm neglected to discuss how important obtaining sexual satisfaction was for women.

Capelle (1993) points out how Thompson was primarily interested in ameliorating suffering. She struggled to find new solutions to the problems women encountered in society. The socialist feminist Sheila Rowbotham (2015) argues that "all revolutionary movements create their own ways of seeing" (p. 28).

Rowbotham reminds us that finding a new consciousness takes time: ". . . the creation of an alternative world and an alternative culture cannot be the work of a day . . . theoretical consistency is difficult . . . often it comes out of dogmatism" (p. 28).

Dogmatism was not Thompson's style. When it comes to the psychology of women, we can marvel at her insights, her radical stance, and at other times be sorely disappointed by her blind spots.

Clara Thompson was not the only woman writing about sexuality. Her colleague and friend Frieda Fromm-Reichmann contributed to the literature as well. Thompson met Frieda Fromm-Reichmann at Baden-Baden in 1927. Silver (1995) provides a richly drawn history about Frieda Fromm-Reichmann drawing our attention to how she wrote about "Female Psychosexuality" (1995) and to her early 1927 essay on "Jewish Food Rituals" first published in German. It was when Fromm-Reichmann moved to Chestnut Lodge that she became close friends with Thompson's analysand Marjorie Jarvis (Hornstein, 2000). Jarvis was divorced and had a daughter who became part of the Chestnut Lodge family. Jarvis and Fromm-Reichmann were frequently sited together and looked "dashing with their matching cigarette holders" (Hornstein, 2000, p. 106). Fromm-Reichmann kept secret that during her medical school training, she was raped (Shapiro, 2002). Hornstein (2002) suggests that the experience influenced her clinical work. Fromm-Reichmann explained that "dissociation of traumatic material" temporarily restricted awareness and was as significant as repression in the case of psychosis. Hornstein points out that Fromm-Reichmann's view was similar to "contemporary concepts of posttraumatic stress and its attendant pathology. (p. 411, n. 4).

During a symposium, Fromm-Reichmann commented on Thompson's paper titled *Cultural Complications in the Sexual life of Women*; she commented that Thompson had said far too little about the significance of the devaluation of women's procreative capacities. There is a "repression" she argued of the fact that "women gain not only spiritual satisfaction but also sexual gratification from carrying a child, from delivering it and from breast feeding it" (Capelle, 1993, p. 381).

As Thompson began to respond to Fromm-Reichmann's criticism, a technical glitch occurred—the recorder broke. Capelle (1993) suggests the glitch is symbolic for the lack of support Thompson received from her colleagues. Fromm-Reichmann like Horney and Deutsch maintained that there were more important problems for women than those Thompson had described.

Capelle (1993) argues that only a few of her many students and analysands "adopted her view" (p. 382) on the issue of women's psychology. Thompson's analysand Ruth Moulton's (1970) essay reflects some of Thompson's views.

> The amount of narcissistic injury connected with the lack of a penis depends in part on its value in a given culture and a specific family. The degree of penis envy experienced will vary according to how the woman has been led to view her own functions, whether as something valuable or as worthless. Clara Thompson pointed out that penis envy is often symbolic of envy of wider aspects of male power and privilege, and is more prevalent in a competitive setting or one where boys are preferred and an inferior evaluation is placed on girls. A comparable phenomenon is seen in men: Those who are insecure about their sexual competence overvalue and envy the size of the penis of father, brother, or other competitor. Thus, both sexes tend to see the penis as a power symbol, apart from its specific functions.
>
> I am suggesting that an evanescent phase of penis envy is apt to occur when the little girl first becomes aware of the existence of a penis. This is in the nature of universal childhood curiosity and interest in anything new and may be quite transitory if she is fairly satisfied with being a girl and has been allowed or encouraged to develop appropriate awareness of her own body function. This awareness is ultimately based on autonomous, internal sensations but consensual validation and affirmation are entailed in its realistic evaluation. If healthy growth ensues, this early, primary type of penis envy may easily pass, causing no significant conflict. It is neither malignant nor a ubiquitous obstacle. On the other hand, it may be secondarily reinforced under certain conditions so that it does become an important facet of a later neurotic problem. Even then, it is part of a process, not the cause.
>
> (p. 90)

Moulton emerges as one of Thompson's students who carried forth her ideas. In "Early Papers on Women: Horney to Thompson" (1975), she concluded that:

> Horney was freer from a strong personal bond to Freud than women who had worked closely with him, such as Helene Deutsch, Jeanne Lampl De Groot, Ruth Mack Brunswick, and Marie Bonaparte. All of these latter women wrote extensively applying Freud's theories to women, carrying out his suggestion that women would have to help solve their own secrets. However, none of them ever really broke away from Freud, and their differences with him were carefully couched in orthodox terminology. Apparently, those who fell under the sway of his great charisma had trouble in getting free of his influence.
>
> (p. 210)

Thompson did not suffer this connection with Freud.

Mary Lou Lionells claims Thompson as her "analytic Grandmother" and speaks to—a proud heritage.[16] She views Thompson as

> Far ahead of her time, Clara Thompson was a feminist who explored cultural expectations of gender differences. She rejected Freudian theory on the basis of its lacking an empathic feminine viewpoint. Her writing on female psychological issues offers insights concerning gender identity, work and motherhood, intimacy, aggressivity and sexuality that remain of value in contemporary psychoanalytic work.
>
> (Lionells, 1995, p. 224)

Touching the Future

Thompson's feminism came of age between the first and second waves of the women's rights movements. She was the product of a feminist generation that advocated for a binary sex equality. She rejected Freud's theory because she could see his masculine bias. Where Freud saw penis envy as the problem, Thompson saw the realistic advantages given to those with a penis. The penis, she argued, was a symbol of inequity. Where Freud argued the best solution for women was to accept their feminine role instead of developing either a neurosis or a masculinity complex, Thompson (1942) refuted these solutions, suggesting instead the "culture invites masculinity in women" (p. 338). She argued,

> However, there are other implications in the idea of accepting the feminine role—it may include the acceptance of the whole group of attitudes considered feminine by the culture at the time. In such a sense acceptance of the feminine role may not be an affirmative attitude at all but an expression of submission and resignation. It may mean choosing the path of least resistance with the sacrifice of important parts of the self for security.
>
> (p. 338)

It took until the 1960s and 1970s feminist movement, particularly the popular book *The Feminine Mystique* (1963), written by the iconic second-wave feminist Betty Friedan, for Thompson's essays on the psychology of women to gain popularity.

> The problem [for women] lay buried, unspoken, for many years in the minds of American women. It was a strange stirring, a sense of dissatisfaction, a yearning [that is, a longing] that women suffered in the middle of the 20th century in the United States. Each suburban [house]wife struggled with it alone. As she made the beds, shopped for groceries . . . she was afraid to ask even of herself the silent question—"Is this all?"
>
> (p. 57)

Of note Betty Freidan's analyst William Menaker, married to Esther Menaker, was in a study group with Thompson in the 1930s. It was Friedan who inserted Thompsonian arguments into popular cultural discourse:

> Women are as capable as men for any type of work or any career path. That put them (women) at odds with the mass media, educators, and psychologists.

In her essays, Thompson was resolute biology did not confer any special qualities. She did not deny the existence of biological differences, but they did not account for inequality. In another time, Thompson might have been drawn to the work of Anne Fausto-Sterling (1985, 2000) for the way she engages the concepts of nature and nurture, as Fausto-Sterling argues it is not an either/or discussion. She claims that society's ideas about male and female are constructed and that we come to view situations based on a complex set of expectations.

In the 1950s, Thompson's work was taken up and used by sociologists who found her ideas about women's psychology and her critique of Freud helpful. However, the support of sociologists may have added fuel to the psychoanalysts who relegated Thompson's work as more sociology than psychoanalysis.

Thompson's essays address the cultural conflicts and double binds that lead to internal struggles for women. She speaks to how a woman must hold in mind two ideas in opposition to each other: self-fulfillment and service to others.

Changing Times

Adrienne Rich (1977) cites Thompson's "early political views on women." Rich's arguments run closer to Thompson's than to Horney's, in her treatise on the bondage of motherhood.

In Thompson's essay "Changing Concepts of Homosexuality in Psychoanalysis" (1947), she shows an evolving awareness of the difference between sex and gender. The essay speaks to the messy way the term "homosexual" has been used in psychoanalysis. ". . . anything which pertains in any way to a relationship, hostile or friendly, to a member of one's own sex may be termed "homosexual." Under these circumstances what does an analyst convey to himself, his audience, or his patient when he says the patient has homosexual trends?"

She poses another interesting question, "[W]hat might happen if a person could continue his development in a culture with no sex restrictions. It is possible that most children would eventually develop a preference for the biologically most satisfactory type of sexual gratification and that that would prove to be found in the union of male and female genitals. If it should be found that heterosexual activity eventually became the preferred form of sex life, would this mean that the other forms had been repressed? If the culture were truly uncriticizing, repression would be unnecessary. . . . In other words, it is probable that on the physiological level uninhibited humans would get their sex gratification in any way possible—but if they had a choice, they would choose the most pleasurable" (p. 184).

Her speculations maintain a heterosexual bias, though she does assume that beyond the biological sex of the individual, a "relationship" with the other person has interpersonal meaning (p. 186). As she opines on gay marriage her ambivalences show through:

> Homosexual marriage, by which I mean a relatively durable, long-term relationship between two people—a relationship in which the interests and personalities of each are important to the other . . . all the pictures of a neurotic heterosexual adult love relationship can exist. Adult love seems to be a rare experience in our culture anyway and would doubtless be even more rare among homosexuals, because a person with the necessary degree of maturity would probably prefer a heterosexual relation unless external circumstances in his life made this impossible . . . even though the specific cause for homosexuality cannot be found, the specific needs which it satisfies can be examined. Obviously, it gives sexual satisfaction and for a person unable to make contact with the opposite sex, this is important . . . also it helps cope with the problem of loneliness and isolation. The very fact of belonging to a culturally taboo group has its satisfactions . . . in no case will it be found to be the cause of the rest of the neurotic structure—the basic origin of the neurosis—although after it is established, it may contribute to the problems . . . psychoanalysis must deal primarily with the personality structure realizing that the symptom is a secondary development from that.
>
> (pp. 188–189)

In 1949, Bertram Schaffner, an openly gay psychoanalyst was in treatment with Thompson, and experienced first-hand her attitudes toward homosexuality he thought,

> harbored the feeling then prevalent, that homosexuality was subject to modification or even reversal as a result of good psychoanalysis . . . this may have led her into being overly trusting of me when I suggested becoming engaged to a remarkable woman I had met . . . apparently, Dr. Thompson failed to grasp my transference to her, i.e., my need to please her (as I would have wanted to please my mother) by getting married.
>
> (Goldman, 1995, p. 249)

Thompson struggled with her ambivalences. She did not pathologize, yet on the topic she was not as progressive as we might wish. Nonetheless, she deserves credit as a 20th-century theorist for struggling to examine, understand, and challenge key concepts that were foundational to her field. Psychoanalysis was still haunted by theories of "hereditary degeneration and neurosis" when it came to same-sex sexualities (Faderman, 1981, p. 239).

Clara Thompson's writing about women and society included insights on gender, work, and motherhood. She explored the issues around intimacy, aggression, and women's sexuality. Her essays remain relevant today. She was working on a book that was to be called *Problems of Womanhood* (Capelle, 1993, p. 382). The book was never completed.

Notes

1 Elizabeth Capelle (1993, 1998) describes the connection between the leadership of the culture-and-personality school anthropologists, Sapir, Benedict, and Mead, with the cultural school of psychoanalysis. From her work we learn that by the turn of the century, the Columbia University scholar Franz Boas was already developing his ideas about cultural anthropology and that it was his students Sapir, Benedict, and Mead who further developed their teacher's ideas about cultural anthropology into a distinctive way of thinking. In her dissertation, Elizabeth Capelle (1993) writes that "in their search for a more satisfactory understanding of the psychological mechanisms of the 'tyranny of culture,' the culture-and-personality anthropologists had begun to investigate psychoanalysis" (1993, p. 245). She notes that

> They found willing collaborators in Harry Stack Sullivan, Karen Horney, Erich Fromm and Clara Thompson, the analysts who were to become known as the "cultural school." The two groups had been brought together through the agencies of Sullivan, who since meeting Sapir in 1926 had been a fervent advocate of interdisciplinary collaboration.
>
> (pp. 247–248)

2 Rubins (1978) p. 250 describes the panel's participants. It included Abe Maslow.
3 This quote is taken from the unpublished paper held in the WAW archives. It was later published in 1943 as "*Penis Envy in Women.*"
4 Horney (1926) argued that Freud had overestimated the notion of penis envy in girls and insisted instead that gender differences were due to the patriarchal culture.
5 See Bacciagaluppi, M. (2001) Fromm's Concern with Feminine Values. *Journal of the American Academy of Psychoanalysis 29*, 617–624.
6 Groddeck was a German physician thought of as the father of somatic medicine. Freud and his followers including Ferenczi, Horney, Fromm and Thompson frequented his spa in Baden-Baden.

7 This was eight years after she first presented her paper on Penis Envy,
8 Symposium was sponsored by the Psychoanalytic Division of the Department of Psychiatry at New York Medical College.
9 See Herschberger, R. (2016) *Sexual differences and character trends*, for a discussion of Fromm's position.
10 See *Juliet Mitchell and Psychoanalytic Feminism*, Nasrullah Mambrol (2016) in *Literary Theory and Criticism*, for a discussion Mitchell's theory. Mambrol, N. (2016, December 16) Juliet Mitchell and Psychoanalytic Feminism. Literary Theory and Criticism. Social Media Site. https://literariness.org/2016/12/13/juliet-mitchell-and-psychoanalytic-feminism
11 I understand there are multiple genders but that was not the language of the time.
12 Moulton (1969) asserts, "During my analytic training I worked with three supervisors, Erich Fromm, Harry Stack Sullivan, and Frieda Fromm-Reichmann, in that order."
13 In the forward to the 1972 edition, Helen Swift Perry claims Clara Thompson told her she wrote the chapter.
14 The psychoanalyst Barbara Waxenberg, a decade or more after Thompson recalled that during her training, she felt the not-so-subtle discrimination in the way the men referred to their female colleagues in training as the "big breasts."
15 This paper was initially presented at a symposium on "Feminine Psychology: Its Implications for Psychoanalytic Medicine" in 1950, was sponsored by the Psychoanalytic Division of the Department of Psychiatry at New York Medical College. Originally titled "Cultural Complications in the Sexual Life of Women," it was ultimately published as "Some Effects of the Derogatory Attitude Towards Female Sexuality" (1950a).

References

See Bacciagaluppi, M. (2001) Fromm's Concern with Feminine Values. *Journal of the American Academy of Psychoanalysis 29*, 617–624.
Benjamin, J. (1988). *The bonds of love: Psychoanalysis, feminism, and the problem of domination*. Pantheon, New York.
Capelle, E. L. (1993). Analyzing the "modern woman": Psychoanalytic debates about feminism, 1920–1950 (Unpublished doctoral dissertation). Columbia University.
Capelle, E. L. (1998). Clara Thompson as culturalist. *Psychoanalytic Review*, *85*(1), 75–93.
Chodorow, N. J. (1978). *The reproduction of mothering: Psychoanalysis and the sociology of gender*. Irvine: University of California Press.
Dimen, M. (1995). The third step: Freud, the feminists, and postmodernism. *American Journal of Psychoanalysis*, *55*(4), 303–319.
Faderman, L. (1981). *Surpassing the love of men*. New York: Women's Press.
Fausto-Sterling, A. (1985). *Myths of gender: Biological theories about women and men*. New York: Basic Books.

Fausto-Sterling, A. (2000). *Sexing the body: Gender politics and the construction of sexuality*. New York: Basic Books.

First, E. (1974, May 19). Psychoanalysis and feminism. *New York Times*, p. 382.

Flax, J. (2002). Resisting woman, *Contemporary Psychoanalysis, 38*(2), 257–276, DOI: 10.1080/00107530.2002.10747100.

Friedan, B. (1963). *The feminine mystique*. New York: W. W. Norton & Company.

Fromm, E. (1943). Sex and character. *Psychiatry, 6*, 22.

Fromm-Reichmann, F. (1995). Female psychosexuality. *Journal of the American Academy of Psychoanalysis, 23*(1), 19–32.

Fromm-Reichmann, F., & Bever, C. T. (1995). Jewish food rituals. *Journal of the American Academy of Psychoanalysis, 23*(1), 7–17.

Gallop, J. (1982). *Feminism and psychoanalysis: The daughter's seduction.* Springer.

Gilligan, C. (1982). *In a different voice: Psychological theory and women's development*. Cambridge, MA: Harvard University Press.

Goldman, S. (1995). The difficulty of being a gay psychoanalyst during the last fifty years: An interview with Dr. Bertram Schaffner. In *Disorienting sexuality: Psychoanalytic reappraisals of sexual identities*. London and New York: Routledge Press.

Green, M. R. (Ed.). (1964). *Interpersonal psychoanalysis: The selected papers of Clara M. Thompson*. New York: Basic Books.

Horney, K. (1926). The flight from womanhood: The masculinity-complex in women, as viewed by men and by women. *International Journal of Psychoanalysis, 7*, 324–339.

Horney, K. (1937). *The neurotic personality of our time*. New York: W. W. Norton & Company.

Horney, K. (1939). *New ways in psychoanalysis*. London: Routledge.

Hornstein, G. (2000). *To redeem one person is to redeem the world: The life of Frieda Fromm-Reichmann*. New York: The Free Press.

Lionells, M. (1995). Interpersonal-relational psychoanalysis: An introduction and overview of contemporary implications and applications. *International Forum of Psychoanalysis, 4*(4), 223–230.

Mitchell, J. (1974). *Psychoanalysis and feminism*. New York: Pantheon.

Mambrol, N. (2016, December 16) Juliet Mitchell and Psychoanalytic Feminism. Literary Theory and Criticism. Social Media Site. https://literariness.org/2016/12/13/julit-mitchell-and-psychoanalytic-feminism/

Moulton, R. (1969). My memories of being supervised. *Contemporary Psychoanalysis, 5*(2), 151–157.

Moulton, R. (1970). A survey and reevaluation of the concept of penis envy. *Contemporary Psychoanalysis, 7*(1), 84–104.

Moulton, R. (1975). Early papers on women: Horney to Thompson. *American Journal of Psychoanalysis, 35*(3), 207–223.

Rich, A. (1977). *Of woman born: Motherhood as experience and institution*. New York: W. W. Norton.

Rowbotham, S. (2015). *Woman's consciousness, man's world*. London: Verso Trade.

Shapiro, S. (2002). The history of feminism and interpersonal psychoanalysis. *Contemporary Psychoanalysis, 38*(2), 213–256.

Silver, A. L. S. (1995). Introduction to Fromm-Reichmann's "female psychosexuality" and "Jewish food rituals." *Journal of the American Academy of Psychoanalysis, 23*(1), 1–6.

Sullivan, H. S. (1965). *Personal psychopathology*. Washington, DC: The William Alanson White Psychiatric Foundation.

Thompson, C. (1937). Sexuality: Karen Horney. [Review of the essay "The problem of feminine masochism" by K. Horney]. *International Journal of Psychoanalysis, 18*, 64–65.

Thompson, C. (1941). The role of women in this culture. *Psychiatry, 4*(1), 1–8.

Thompson, C. (1942). Cultural pressures in the psychology of women. *Psychiatry, 5*(3), 331–339.

Thompson, C. (1942, May 19) What is penis envy? (Conference presentation) *The Annual Convention of the Association for the Advancement of Psychoanalysis in Boston*, MA.

Thompson, C. (1943). "Penis envy" in women. *Psychiatry, 6*(2), 123–125.

Thompson, C. (1947). Changing concepts of homosexuality in psychoanalysis. *Psychiatry, 10*, 183–189.

Thompson, C. (1950a). Some effects of the derogatory attitude towards female sexuality. *Psychiatry, 13*(3), 349–354.

Thompson, C. (1950b, March 18). Cultural complications in the sexual life of woman. In *Feminine psychology: Its implications for psychoanalytic medicine. Symposium proceedings* (Vol. 19) Department of Psychiatry NY Medical College. New York.

Thompson, C. (1964). The interpersonal approach to the clinical problems of masochism. In M. R. Green (Ed.), *Interpersonal psychoanalysis: The selected papers of Clara M. Thompson* (pp. 183–198). New York: Basic Books.

Wake, N. (2011). *Private practices: Harry Stack Sullivan, the science of homosexuality, and American liberalism*. New Brunswick, NJ: Rutgers University Press.

Chapter 6

The William Alanson White Institute

"It's My Child"[1]

Clara Thompson served as the Director of the William Alanson White Institute (WAWI) from 1946 until her death in 1958. Being the Director of WAWI was deeply pleasing to Thompson who found it "a tribute" to her leadership abilities. With that title, Green (1964) writes, she, "dedicated herself even more zealously to this small band of pioneers" (p. 355). The band of pioneers included the founders Erich Fromm, Frieda Fromm-Reichmann, Harry Stack Sullivan, David Rioch, Janet M. Rioch, and their students who had left the Horney institute in the walkout of 1941. Thompson fought many battles to both attain and hold on to her position during the 12 years between her appointment as Director and President of the Board Trustees in 1946 and her death in 1958. Those years were marked by clashes for control over who should be trained as a psychoanalyst and who should train them, as well as the broader question of what constitutes and is entitled to be called psychoanalysis. One dispute present from the onset concerned who would be trained at WAWI. The training of non-medical psychoanalysts (mainly PhD psychologists) was a stormy issue in the wider world of American psychoanalysis. Erich Fromm, a founding member, had earlier been denied the title of training analyst at the Association for the Advancement of Psychoanalysis because he was a non-medically trained clinician. He held the distinction of being the only non-physician founding member at WAWI, ensuring the issue stayed in the forefront of organizational discussions.

How did Clara Thompson achieve her position? The road to becoming Director was both visionary and complicated. It would be fair to say it began in 1930 when Thompson was made the first President of the Washington-Baltimore Psychoanalytic Society. In 1933, when she returned from Budapest and moved to New York she renewed her in-person association

DOI: 10.4324/9781003284840-7

with the Washington-Baltimore Psychoanalytic Society. Kwawer (2019) provides some details,

> Although Clara Thompson moved to New York City in 1933 after Ferenczi died, she continued to conduct seminars and to offer supervision in Washington, DC. Sullivan remained actively involved in the training activities of the Washington-Baltimore Society, where he and Thompson were both training analysts through the 1930s and 1940s, serving as a member of its Education Committee from 1933 to 1937.
>
> (pp. 86–98)

The Washington-Baltimore Psychoanalytic Society became a formal training program in 1932 and the fourth psychoanalytic society in the United States. It was admitted into the International Psychoanalytic Association (IPA) at the controversial 1932 Wiesbaden meeting, where Thompson was present and where Ferenczi presented his paper, *Confusion of Tongues*. The training program was established a year after the New York Psychoanalytic Institute and simultaneously with institutes in Chicago, and Boston (Kwawer, 2019).

In 1933, Harry Stack Sullivan, along with Edward Sapir and Harold Lasswell, established The William Alanson White Foundation. The Foundation became a base for Sullivan's "major creative activities—especially the Washington School of Psychiatry and the journal *Psychiatry* (Perry, 1982, p. 356). Earlier, as founding members of the Washington-Baltimore Psychoanalytic Society, both Thompson and Sullivan had welcomed "non-medical clinicians" to their developing interdisciplinary perspective (Kwawer, 2019, p. 88).

Sullivan and Thompson worked closely together to establish themselves and to train analysts in a non-Freudian approach to psychoanalysis. But Sullivan's presence was not always an asset. Lewis Hill, a psychiatrist and analysand of Thompson's, became the Director of the Washington-Baltimore Psychoanalytic Institute. He advised Thompson, (in a letter dated January 8, 1941, courtesy of WAWI),

> It might be well to keep H.S.S. as a silent partner in your plans because I think that a good many of the old-guard regard him as a wily rebel who has already cost the Association a good bit in the way of legal expense incurred in developing a constitution which would work.

Lewis's letter calls her attention to the bylaws of the American Psychoanalytic Association of 1941, Vol 1, Article II, Section II, which state:

> No individual member of this Association shall be a member of more
> than one of the societies which are constituent society-members of this
> Association. In the future, in any one locality, sole jurisdiction over
> practice and training shall reside in only one constituent society and
> its institute.

It took a decade to conclude that The American [APsaA] was in violation
of anti-trust laws established to prevent monopolies and prevent harmful
business practices.

Meanwhile, as previously recounted, a second break-up was underway
when in 1943 Karen Horney denied Erich Fromm[2] analytic training rights
at the Association for the Advancement of Psychoanalysis using similar tactics to those used against her when she had been penalized by the New York
Psychoanalytic Institute. Clara Thompson and Harry Stack Sullivan resigned
in support of Erich Fromm and left the Association for the Advancement of
Psychoanalysis. Thompson, Sullivan, and others moved to establish a new
institute that was conceptualized as a New York arm of the Washington
School of Psychiatry with both a Washington and New York Branch. Perry
(1984) notes that these plans were helped by Janet MacKenzie Rioch, "a
close friend and colleague of Thompson's," and her brother David McK.
Rioch, a research scientist and neurophysiologist. (pp. 389–390)

During the following years

> Thompson, Sullivan, Fromm-Reichmann traveled back and forth by
> train between the two cities on a weekly basis. Others, like David
> Rioch and Erich Fromm, came and went less frequently. . . . A wide
> range of students were accepted, and the School became the training
> institute for the Foundation.
>
> (Perry, 1984, p. 390)

Between 1943 and 1947, The Washington-Baltimore Psychoanalytic Society and the Washington School of Psychiatry appeared as one entity; they
shared faculty and maintained joint affiliations.

Then in what Perry (1984) calls "a strange bureaucratic twist," courses
appeared then disappeared in the catalog of the Washington-Baltimore

Psychoanalytic Institute (Society). (p. 391) During this time, the G.I. Bill of Rights introduced a funding stream that would cover expenses to train physicians who were military veterans in psychoanalysis and only the Washington School of Psychiatry qualified for the funding, so the school pulled away from the Washington-Baltimore Psychoanalytic Institute (Society).

Rose Spiegel (1987) reminisced about these days:

> My first days of reaching out coincide with the very first days of the founding of the institute. I am fortunate to have found Clara Thompson in the 1940s when I sought psychoanalysis for my private needs, for what I was then frozen confronting my life. . . . What I was then, and still am impressed with, some forty years later, is the clarity, the decisiveness, and the resourcefulness of their <u>action</u> in the <u>separation</u> and the founding of the White Institute. Imagine, still in the years of the Second World War, they arranged for an exchange commute between Baltimore—Washington and New York, of Sullivan, <u>Frieda Fromm-Reichmann</u>, David Rioch, coming to New York, every three weeks, with Clara, Janet, and Erich taking the teaching trips to Chestnut Lodge. And so, the Institute in the making could have regular lectures and could provide supervision for the fledgling analysts. In 1943, we were the New York Branch of the Washington- Baltimore Psychoanalytic Institute. At that time, we met in Clara's apartment.
>
> (p. 2)

Ruth Moulton (1969), recalled that in the early days (1943–46) at WAWI:

> There were no formal training rules or regulations, nor was there any need for them. Everyone seemed to sense what was going on with everyone else. It was clear from my analysis that Clara Thompson knew what all my supervisors thought about my work. . . . The hours of supervision required were the same as now, but there were fewer courses. The faculty was much smaller, but this was offset by the fact that its members were much more accessible. Training in those years was much more individualized and intimate than possible now, largely because the students and faculty have increased at least five-fold.
>
> The sense of dedication to a liberal analytic cause, and a strong need to prove one's capacity to survive prejudice and isolation, united the

students and faculty. There was also a strong sense of dedication to the intensive treatment of individual patients, with fewer distractions and less external pressure than we all suffer from currently. Thus, one tends to look back with nostalgia on the spirit of those early years when we were the New York Branch of the Washington School of Psychiatry.

(p. 157)

In 1946, the New York branch of the Washington School of Psychiatry became incorporated as the WAWI, making it also eligible for GI benefits. It was then that Clara Thompson became the first Director. Her colleagues, Harry Stack Sullivan and Frieda Fromm-Reichmann kept up their involvement by traveling back and forth between Washington and New York.

WAWI

"WAW [sic] fashioned itself alone in the field among psychoanalytic institutes because they taught more eclectic and, considered, non-Freudian methods of therapy" (Moulton, 1969, p. 157). According to Moulton, students and faculty who helped found the Institute were kept together by "a strong need to prove one's capacity to survive prejudice and isolation" (p. 157).

These early leaders chose Thompson as their director with the goal of promoting a new model of psychoanalysis. Their vision, much like Thompson's youthful desire to become a medical missionary, had the aim of relieving human suffering. Her work with Sándor Ferenczi provided her with a new perspective on psychoanalytic treatment that was warmer, empathic, engaged, and more spontaneous than the orthodox Freudian practices of a blank screen analyst and drive theories. Freud's classical theories and techniques were being reevaluated shifting, as Thompson explains it, to concentrating on finding "more effective methods of therapy and on trying to enlarge the therapeutic scope of psychoanalysis" (Thompson, 1950, p. 5).

Thompson describes a move away from eliminating infantile amnesia toward an understanding of the complicated dynamics of the doctor–patient relationship. This she said, incorporated "Sullivan's theory of interpersonal relations" with "a study of comparative cultures" as the "cultural school of analysts" (Thompson, 1946, p. 5).

As Director, Thompson navigated organizational storms, strategizing and intervening to maintain people on course and steering discussions in her preferred direction. She was adept at identifying her adversaries and keeping them and her allies close. Despite her solid leadership skills and her early support and enthusiasm from the majority of faculty and students, by 1956 tensions were high. Green (1964) reports that she was attacked by some who called her a "matriarchal, subtly dominating woman." Worse, some colleagues saw her as someone "who needed to mother the institute because she was too neurotic to have a life of her own" (Green, 1964, p. 374). These attacks no doubt deepened the wounds of her personal losses, that is, the death of Henry Major in 1948, Harry Stack Sullivan in 1949, and Erich Fromm's move to Mexico in 1949. Sullivan's death in 1949 also dealt a blow to the new organization.[3] The world of New York organizational psychoanalysis was deep in competition, greed, and the need for power, turning disputes into outright wars (Frosch, 1991).

> After Sullivan's death, the American Psychoanalytic Association renewed its attack on the so-called deviationists in both schools. In New York, students were threatened with permanent discrediting if they did not immediately sever all course work and analytic training with the disfavored teachers. This threat was in fact a violation of the antitrust laws and, upon legal advice, was shortly withdrawn.
>
> (p. 391)

Thompson's correspondence with Edward Bibring and Ernest Hadley (Oskar Diethelm Library, Ralph Crowley Papers) depicts a specific conflict that played out following the loss of Sullivan:

May 16, 1950
Dear Dr. Bibring
    Last Saturday I was in Washington and talked with Dr. Hadley and some others in the Washington Society about our status, and I find certain aspects of our relationship to the Washington-Baltimore Institute and the American Psychoanalytic Association are still obscure to the Washington group as well as to those of us in New York . . .
    (1). We have been informed that those of us in New York who have been training and supervising analysts of the Washington-Baltimore Institute for many years may no longer have this title this is confusing

on two scores. (a) What does this mean about our future status if we should become connected with another recognized psychoanalytic Institute? Is our status then automatically reinstated? You probably already have some precedent for this as, for example, Grace Baker, recently of Baltimore, who, I believe is now a training analyst with the Columbia group. Are Dr. Rioch and I to assume that our status as training and supervising analyst in general is not in question and that we can receive such status in some other Institute at anytime as Dr. Baker has? (b) Also how does this loss of status as training analyst affect our relations (specifically those of Dr. Janet Rioch and myself) to the students we are currently supervising in Washington? I am leaving out of consideration our New York program for the sake of simplification. Is it the decision of the American Psychoanalytic Association that any students currently being supervised by us in Washington may no longer receive credit for their supervision? Dr. Hadley is of the opinion and believes we should stop all supervision of students in Washington. Dr. Rioch and I, as well as some others in Washington, are puzzled as to what is the basis of discontinuing our training status in Washington since we are still members in good standing there. This definitely implies some criticism of our competence and can hurt us professionally. Will you please clarify this for us and Dr. Hadley.

(2) The second point is perhaps more important in terms of public relations. A number of the students of the William Allison White Institute of Psychiatry have been registered as students of the Washington-Baltimore Institute for several years. They have paid registration fees and annual dues as students. These checks have been accepted by the Washington-Baltimore Institute. Moreover, our courses have been published for the last three years in the bulletin of the Washington-Baltimore Institute and recognized as training courses. Students have registered with us in good faith on that basis. In other words, a contract exists between some students in our Institute and the Washington-Baltimore Institute. Dr. Hadley feels he cannot answer how the Washington-Baltimore Institute can discharge its legal obligation to our students and he would like you to advise us and him. I do not understand how the Baltimore Division can with any justification disclaim knowledge of what has been going on or disclaim a part of the joint responsibility since there was

nothing secret in the matter. As I said, our courses were announced quite openly in the bulletin and there is no doubt that we are justified in the assumption that the Baltimore Division, by failing to object, tacitly approved. We of course are not seeking to make trouble and we believe these problems can be solved with justice for all. I expect to sail for Europe on May 30th. An answer before that date does not give you much time to consider these matters but I would appreciate it greatly if you could bring some light into this confusion, because the present situation is harmful not only to us but to the good name of the Washington-Baltimore Institute. Sorry to have to continue your "headache."

Sincerely yours, Clara Thompson, Executive Director. Copy to Dr. Hadley

The next day, Ernest Hadley writes to Edward Bibring and includes a copy of Thompson's May 16 letter:

May 17, 1950,
Dear Edward

As you advised me, we dropped the status of teaching, training and supervisor analyst from the end of this teaching season in the case of Clara Thompson, Janet Rioch, Ralph Crowley and Erich Fromm.

Clara seemed quite upset by this.

From her letter to you under date of 16 May, her attitude is improved but continues somewhat rebellious.

I believe my explanation to her was eminently clear on the basis of your advice in December 1949—that it would now be "illegal" to carry them any further.

Enclosed is a proposed page for our forthcoming bulletin. Please advise me if the statement regarding the withdrawal of these names from the list is okay.

As Always, Ernest Hadley, M.D.

The page from the bulletin notes:

Ralph Crowley, M.D. Erich Fromm, Ph.D., Janet MacKenzie Rioch, M.D., and Clara Thompson, M.D. members of the Washington Psychoanalytic Society residing in New York City are being dropped from the list of Training Analysts. They have filed an application for separate Institute status in New York City.

Bibring then writes a two-page letter to Thompson outlining the difficulties:

May 18, 1950
Dear Dr. Thompson
    As anticipated, it is very difficult for me to answer your letter of the of May 16th right now it may take some time to clarify the "confusion" and I certainly cannot do it without consulting the other members of the committee on Institution. The prayers at the president you are referring to seem even more confused since Dr. Grace Baker does not appear on any list of the training analysts we have received during the last year. I am sorry that I cannot be of any help before you sail for Europe, but I shall try to do my best in speeding up the process of clarification.

He asks nine questions including, "How many students do you have in training for psychoanalysis at present? How many students graduated during the last year (1948–1949)?" He questions the connection between the William Alanson White Institute of Psychiatry in New York and the William Alanson White Institute of Psychiatry in Washington. He closes by indicating he is sending a copy of the "recommendations of the Committee on Institutions to the Board of Professional Standards as adopted by the Board at the June 27 meeting in Detroit and the recommendation referring to her application."
    What Bibring does not say is that he was personally responsible for the order for her and others to be dropped from the roster. The lack of transparency made the situation more confusing. Thompson saw through this. On May 29, 1950, Thompson replied:

May 29, 1950
Dear Dr. Bibring
    Thank you for your letter and also for the carbon of the letter to Dr. Hadley. Especially the letter to Dr. Hadley and his reply have clarified for us at least in what direction the main source of our difficulty lies. It is apparently not, as we feared, that the American feels it should offer some sort of punishment by depriving us of training analyst status because, although in good faith but apparently irregularly, we have been carrying on training activities, but the depriving us of the

privilege of training activity in Washington is rather the result of personal hostilities against us within the Washington- Baltimore Institute itself. This unfortunately is an old story in psychoanalytic societies.

However, I shall like to add one or two facts which I find difficult to reconcile with Dr. Hadley's statement that "the names of these analysts (the training analysts in New York) were carried on the list of the Washington division without the consideration of the wishes of the Baltimore division." In the case of at least two of us I do not see how this applies. I was a training analyst of the Washington-Baltimore Society from the day of its birth. Dr. Crowley was a supervising analyst before he left Washington and was later approved as a full training analyst before the Washington-Baltimore Society divided. I believe Dr. Janet Rioch was also accepted before the division. So at the time, at least theoretically, the Baltimore contingent had every opportunity to express dissatisfaction, if such existed, quite openly. That they did not express it openly but actually endorsed the program can be demonstrated by the fact that in the year 1944 or 1945 or part or both, I am not sure of my dates, one student from Baltimore came regularly to Washington for supervision with me when I went down. He did not do this secretly but on the advice and approval of his analyst. I will furnish his name if desired. At that time it was known perfectly definitely by the Baltimore members as well as the Washington members what was going on in New York.

It may be that in the last two or three years the Baltimore Society has had a change of heart and regrets its former cooperation with the Washington Society. Even so I think the depriving of an established training analyst of his rights to train students in the city where he has been recognized as unpleasant implications of incompetence or moral turpitude. Probably this is not worth bothering about. It only concerns us if this action of the Washington-Baltimore Institute would be considered by the APA prejudicial to our becoming recognized as training analysts of the William Alanson White Institute when it is accepted by the American Psychoanalytic Association. I judged from your letter to Dr. Hadley that no such move is contemplated as far as you know.

I am appending the answers to your questions on a separate sheet.
Sincerely yours,
Clara Thompson

At that time, Ernest E. Hadley was Director of the Washington-Baltimore Institute and Lewis B. Hill was the Senior Advisor. It no doubt complicated matters that Lewis Hill was Thompson's former analysand.

Thompson and Fromm Correspondence, 1956–1957

Clara Thompson and Erich Fromm frequently exchanged letters following his move to Mexico in 1949. The letters are filled with personal and professional news. Their correspondence provides a sense of the level of organizational discord as well as the demands placed on Thompson as WAWI's Director. Fromm served as Chairman of the Faculty and Chairman of the Training Committee from 1946 to 1950. He was also the clinical director, a supervisor, and seminar leader (Landis & Tauber, 1971).

Excerpts from a series of letters beginning April 2, 1956, through November 24, 1957 (courtesy of Dr. Ranier Funk, the Erich Fromm Archive, Tubingen) speak to the layers of organizational conflicts. The letters expose both Thompson's vulnerability and her strengths. In the letters, Fromm is heard as her steadfast advocate and at times frank critic. He was her organizational consultant and collaborating partner, her psychoanalyst, and her friend. They plotted together against orthodoxy in whatever form it appeared.

Thompson handled many important issues; she opened the doors to non-psychiatrists for psychoanalytic training and contested the politics of American psychoanalysis. She advocated for the training of psychologists and other professionals and found not only support from Fromm but a colleague in arms. Fromm wanted her alongside him in his effort to keep psychoanalysis from becoming a political tool of orthodoxy. They each wanted psychoanalysis to be a field where creativity would flourish and where psychological research could help to define its mission. While Thompson sought Fromm's counsel, she also held her own opinions. They were respectful and frank with one another as they discussed people and politics.

The letters between Fromm and Thompson are a critical source of biographical information but as Friedman (2013) explains, "at the time of his death, he [Fromm] wanted his wife to destroy all of his letters" (p. xxvii). After persuasive arguments by Rainer Funk, his then research assistant and now literary executor, Fromm allowed Funk to archive his letters. They are now part of the Rainer Funk, Erich Fromm Archive in Tubingen,

Germany, and can be made available with the permission of Rainer Funk who has graciously shared these letters for research purposes and has permitted quotes from certain letters.

By the mid-1950s, Thompson had grown weary. She had struggled with the American for four years trying to gain acceptance for the WAWI. She wrote to Fromm in a letter dated March 11, 1956,[4] that she was "tired" of organizational battles.

David Levy, a vocal psychiatrist at WAWI, was opposed to psychologists becoming equal partners. Ironically, Levy wrote about sibling rivalry and seems to have missed the connection between the battle for status. At the time, psychiatrists feared that psychologists would threaten their livelihood and devalue their status. Fromm and Thompson held a different more inclusive view. Both Fromm and Thompson's intellectual and political liberalism helped fuel the movement away from orthodoxy. Fromm lent Thompson support in her role as Director. Although Thompson split with orthodox psychoanalysis, she knew that the ideas of classical psychoanalysis remained prevalent in the community.

Factions threatened and Thompson's attempts at organizational compromises did not quash the rise of opportunism. She came to realize that she was fighting these organizational battles for herself and her own beliefs.

Fromm, in his letter to Thompson dated March 15, 1956,[5] notes he saw "a real change going on in you, which I hope will continue and make you feel better increasingly." He saw a change both in what she said "directly" and "in your approach to things going on in the Institute." He felt that the "disappearance, or at least decreasing ambivalence" toward him "was an important step forward."

This letter is important as it gives a sense of the politics Thompson had to navigate and the exhaustion that resulted from these multiple battles. Fromm's observation tells us something of Thompson's psychoanalytic treatment. It may have been initially difficult for her to relate to him as her analyst, given her lingering attachment to Ferenczi. Her resistance in her subsequent analysis is understandable. She loved Ferenczi for his warm acceptance and care. As she revealed in her interview with Eissler, mourning Ferenczi's death was difficult, she couldn't say goodbye. But she knew she needed to move on. She came to have a deep abiding respect for Erich Fromm. Their analytic relationship was not built on Thompson's early dependency needs as it was in her treatment with Ferenczi but on her need for independence and respect. One might say with Ferenczi she found her voice and with Fromm she learned how to use it.

Erich Fromm was ahead of his time in understanding the damage of authoritarianism on society and psychoanalysis (Fromm, 1958). As he cautioned Thompson about institutional fights, his intellectual brilliance shines through in his understanding of democracy and the anti-democratic character of traditional psychoanalysis. He warns that they are both "ugly" and the latter prevented "doing really good work with students."[6]

Fromm also identified the power struggle aimed at taking over the Institute and voiced his anger. Thompson's capacity to suppress her anger may have endeared her to people, more so than Fromm, and certainly more than Sullivan and Horney. In the organizational politics of psychoanalysis that may have been an asset in her leadership role. However, she may have had earlier success in admitting non-medical professionals for training if she had been more forceful.

It was Fromm who described how the psychoanalytic institution came with an authoritarian aspect that explained why the field was unwelcoming to dissidents no matter how close they had been to Freud (e.g. Rank and Ferenczi). For her part, Thompson brought a steady hand to the organization and a nascent gender analysis that also addressed the competition between women and men in the business and professional world (Thompson, 1942). In a letter Thompson wrote to Fromm on April 2, 1956, she discloses how she was "impressed" with her, "increased ability to stand stress since the great Horney split in 1942." She adds, "For a little frightened child in a hostile world I am not doing so badly—if you take any satisfaction in your products." The last line refers to her analysis with Fromm.

She shared with Fromm the specific characters and details fueling the disputes at WAWI. One came in a 1956 petition by a group of WAWI analysts to unseat her as director for her views on training non-medical individuals. Thompson claimed that their petition was filled with misstatements about the battle between psychologists and psychiatrists. She thought the entire issue was used to deflect from the dissatisfactions at the Institute that centered on the differences between the more orthodox analysts and those like her who held more liberal views of the field. She concludes in the April 2, 1956 letter,

> You know it's interesting—personal attacks on me do not upset me but I have a real stake in the survival of the institute. Is that neurotic?

> Do I care too much? I asked myself. Obviously I can survive without it but life would be emptier somehow. That's the trouble. It is my child.

The letter is poignant. She characterizes her attachment to the institute as her "child," a sentiment that speaks to the weight as well as the joy she experienced as its Director. In her 1958 essay, Thompson warned psychoanalytic candidates against thinking of an institute as their home, yet she did not heed her own warning. Like everybody else, she lived with her own contradictions. Sometimes it led to mistakes. Fromm did not hold back his criticism. In a letter dated April 3, 1956,[7] Fromm writes to Thompson saying,

> I think you made a mistake in the first place to set it up [WAWI] the way you did. You gave up the psychologists in order to win the favor of Rado, Levy and so on. . . . I think the mistake was that the new organization was already beginning in this way with compromises and opportunism.

Fromm's framework for organizational psychoanalysis was interdisciplinary. He believed that all psychoanalytic work must include the study of the unconscious.

Thompson believed she was gaining ground at WAWI. Her supporters far outnumbered those who signed the petition against her. The make-up of the membership at the Institute was changing, leaning more in her direction. Still there were missteps.

An example is heard in her letter to Fromm dated April 8, 1956,[8] where she identifies her supporters and names one as Abram Kardiner. She writes, "Kardiner is with us as much as he can be counted on. I suspect it is because he wants us to train his wife as a lay analyst. Self-interest seems to be the great legitimate motive today."

However, Kardiner, who she thought was possibly on her side, was most clearly not progressive. Kardiner's two-part essay, "The Social Distress Syndrome of Our Time" (1978), is a clear treatise against liberalism.[9]

She writes in her letter to Fromm dated April 8, 1956[10]

> My hope & belief is that no immediate action will be taken by the Fellows but a committee will be appointed to work on improvements,

when some of the heat & mudslinging lies down perhaps something good will emerge. It has made me think a great deal about the future of the institute. We had some pretty creative talent to begin with— you, Harry Stack & Frieda. I am really distressed by the lack of talent in the present group.

Thompson, now acutely aware of the political hazards in organizations, was growing tired. While Fromm encouraged her to join him in establishing a new national organization, she was disinterested in beginning anew. She tells Fromm in the April 8, 1956, letter that she learned from the experience of forming WAWI that,

what happens as soon as an organization begins to form, vested interests move in & the organization becomes a power tool & its other functions become secondary.

She was feeling nostalgic for the past when she had both the support and creative energy of her colleagues. While her energy was running low, Fromm was still energized and willing to mobilize and begin a new organization if necessary.

In his letter to Thompson on April 12, 1956,[11] he takes issue with her assessment of the situation and asks the quintessential question about the resolution of the fight over training psychologists, "Does that mean those for continuation of the training of psychologists were in the majority?" Fromm was motivated to continue to fight conservatism and thinks Thompson is not radical enough. He tells her,

I think you make one mistake. You still do not sufficiently appreciate the connection between character and theoretical productiveness.

His position is firm "it is only to a certain extent that theoretical creativeness is the result of talent." For Fromm it is more "a matter of character, of courage and of integrity, of being able to see things clearly and to penetrate the surface of public opinion and common sense."

He reprimands Thompson,

I think you fall for a compromise position.

The real question is whether we find satisfaction in a productive effort in life, that is, in genuine interest, productiveness, love, etc., or want satisfaction in prestige and status because one does not exercise one's productive powers. You know that, and yet you are impressed again and again with the opposite standpoint, and tend to make compromises in your own mind, and also practically.

Fromm wanted Thompson to make a clear case for allowing psychologists to be trained. He warned her that if she did not, "The result will only be that the fight goes underground, and sterility will occur."

Fromm makes the case that problems with power develop in organizations because of the character of the people in them. He argues, "I think it would have been much better if you had not accepted the condition of the exclusion of psychologists, and if you had taken the lead yourself."

Thompson does not become defensive. Instead, she utilizes Fromm's criticisms. In her letter to Fromm on May 4, 1956,[12] she reports on progress at the Institute. Both she and Ed Tauber wanted to continue to train psychologists. A new society, the Academy of Psychoanalysis, had agreed to create a new category for non-medical analysts—she reports to Fromm they will be, "honorary & associates, the latter will consist of psychiatrists, social science anthropologists etc. who are contributing to the field of psychoanalysis, so they are there on paper—whether any of them ever get elected is another matter."

By early fall Thompson knew she had cancer, but she remained optimistic. On October 8, 1956, in a letter to Fromm,[13] she shared her medical news and added news of an organizational triumph.

> In [an] "unequivocal statement" "we approved the principle of the training of psychologists permanently by the institute."

A month later, in her letter to Fromm dated November 24, 1956,[14] Thompson lets Fromm know she wants to live. She had been free from illness for most of her life except for having typhoid fever when she was at Phipps and what later may have been a case of endocarditis. Now she felt the surgery for her cancer was curative and was feeling hopeful. Sadly, that would not last long.

Thompson as Leader

Thompson gave birth to the Interpersonal tradition as it was practiced at WAWI. Listening to her introductory remarks as the first President of the Board of Trustees of WAW Institute of Psychiatry, we hear her in action:

> Tonight, the William Alanson White Institute of Psychiatry holds its first public lecture as an independent Institute. In December 1933, largely at the instigation of Dr. Sullivan, seconded and approved by Dr. White, the William Alanson White Psychiatric Foundation was incorporated in Washington. Its aim was to bring psychiatry in the social sciences together for the purpose of research into the human personality. To accomplish this Dr. Sullivan recommended that psychiatry should be given the opportunity to profit by the work of the social sciences and in turn, the social sciences should be enriched by education in psychiatric principles.
>
> (Thompson, 1938, p. 1)

> To further their approach, the Washington School of Psychiatry was established in 1936 as a project of the William Alanson White Foundation. For several years, the school functioned only in Washington. However, in May 1943, under pressure of wartime needs and an increased demand for psychiatric training from members of various professions, it was decided to enlarge the scope of the school and to establish a division in New York City.

In this introduction, Thompson provides a history of the Institute without articulating her role in its development. Since she felt the Institute was her "child," we would expect to hear her parental role in her reflections. A change in tone occurs when she speaks to the history starting in 1946, when she became the Institute Director. Her syntax changes, she uses the pronouns "we" and "our," and in that subtle switch, she claims ownership.

> The New York Division rapidly increased in size, and in 1946, in order to be chartered under the Board of Regents and the State of New York, a separate corporation was formed which took its name as The William Alanson White Institute of Psychiatry. Under this name, *we* have had a charter as an educational institution since October 1946. Although *we* have changed *our* name, in most important respects *we* have not essentially changed our relation to the Washington School of Psychiatry. *We* are still closely connected in *our* teaching staff, program, interest, and aims.

Our Institute at the present time offers two types of graduate training. *We* offer comprehensive training to psychiatrists in the theory and practice of psychoanalysis. True to Dr. White's vision, *we* place special emphasis on the relation of personality problems to culture, and *our* students have the opportunity to become acquainted with the social sciences.

We also provide psychoanalytic orientation to selected professional workers in allied fields, such as medicine, the social sciences, psychology, social work, teaching, and the ministry.

The whole spirit and plan of *our* school was inspired by the vision and active interest of the late William Alanson White, for many years the head of St. Elizabeth's Hospital in Washington, DC. Under his influence, the hospital became one of the foremost institutions for research in and therapy for mental disorder. . . . Dr. Sullivan and *I* both had the fortunate experience of working under Dr. White's direction at St. Elizabeths Hospital around 1920. *I* am sure Dr. Sullivan will agree with *me* that he had the quality, all too rare in great thinkers, of inspiring and appreciating the development of those working with him. His interests were not merely limited to hospital problems. He saw psychiatry as having a role to play in the social order, a role greater than the mere care for the mentally ill. He felt the social sciences should collaborate with medicine in seeking the causes of mental disorder in society . . .

So *we* are proud to have *our* Institute bear the name of this pioneer psychiatrist. The roots of *our* work are in his thinking, and *we* believe our aims and goals are extensions and outgrowths of this own.

In presenting *our* Institute for the first time officially to the public, *we* have chosen as *our* speaker Dr. Harry Stack Sullivan, the founder of the William Alanson White Foundation, a friend and collaborator of Dr. White. Dr. Sullivan, whose researches in schizophrenia and whose book *Conceptions of Modern Psychiatry* are well known to many of you, will speak tonight on "The Meaning of Anxiety in Psychiatry and in Life.

Thompson commands the helm as she provides a thumbnail sketch of this important history. She divides the source of developmental energy between Harry Stack Sullivan and William Alanson White. But by her subtle and consistent use of the pronoun "we" as the speaker, she places herself together with Sullivan and White. She takes ownership when she uses "our" to indicate belonging, and she ends by signaling with her *we* that she has invited Sullivan to give a paper in her institute.

This style is on view again 20 years later when she delivers the Harry Stack Sullivan Society lecture titled "The History of the William Alanson White Institute" (March 15, 1955). She begins this talk by alerting her audience that her "compulsive modesty" was disturbed when she realized she had chosen such a big title. She claims to have done so "absent-mindedly" (Thompson, 2017, p. 7). This is characteristic of Thompson. She backs away from owning the magnitude of her statements as she forges ahead. Her suggestion that she was somehow distracted when she chose the title is meant to disarm. Old patterns die hard. There are remnants of the dutiful child of her youth, who defensively tried to hide her real feelings to not disturb her mother. Now it's her colleagues she does not want to upset. What she has to say, however, is not at all hesitant; she goes right to the core of psychoanalytic disputes and brings up sexuality immediately by invoking the idea of incest.

> I think psychoanalysis is an unusually incestuous specialty. The father-son situation or the mother-son situation is very strong in our whole field and the difficulty that sons have had getting free from these fathers has punctuated the whole history of psychoanalysis. Either the tendency is to submit and be a good son or be rebellious. Now, these rebellious sons have been told so in just so many terms many times, and Freud was the one who started this insidious custom. I am sure you have read enough of the literature to know that when Adler disagreed with him, he said that Adler's difficulty was that he was a short man; therefore he had an inferiority feeling; therefore he had to have power. In other words, he borrowed Adler's theory to squelch him. When Jung decided to desexualize the libido theory, he told Jung that the trouble with him was his Protestant-Puritanism. When Ferenczi decided that it was a good idea to like our patients, Freud told him he was in his second childhood and that what was the matter with him was that he wanted love himself.
>
> (p. 8)

Disagreeing with Freud was dangerous. He was likely to distract from the core of his critic's arguments with personalized attacks. Thompson keenly aware of this trend in psychoanalysis was mindful of how dissenters were silenced.

Her lack of arrogance was a personality characteristic that helped her navigate treacherous turf. She softly wore the mantle of executive and chief while she rose to the top of her field. It was not a matter of meekness but of integrity. At times she reverted to a defensive style, disguising her true feelings to disarm the other. This style turned into an effective leadership tool. While she was forthright in her opinions, she could arrive through the back door without ruffling her opponents' feathers. In that way, she could be called cunning or as Sullivan named her, a "puma." She also did not want to repeat the mistakes of the men around her—not because she saw herself as better but because she saw that path as misguided and dangerous. Sullivan had followers but also made enemies; Fromm's confrontational style offended people. Thompson was best suited for the job. Fromm (Green, 1964) noted that Thompson "guided the students and colleagues, with great patience, and with remarkable modesty." These qualities he felt "made it possible for her to lead the institute without ever permitting it to become the center of a "school" in which one special theory was taught as the right and orthodox one" (vi).

Thompson's style was one of sincere collaboration and coalition building. As she said in *Psychoanalysis: Evolution and Development* (1950):

> Psychoanalysis did not spring full grown from the brow of Freud. It has a history. Nor has there been a straight line of development. Since it evolved under the stress of practical exigencies, it shows gaps, regressions, by-paths, as well as progressions.
>
> (p. v)

The evolution of Thompson's psychoanalytic theories is similar. They wind and weave together different ideas of Freud, Ferenczi, Horney, Sullivan, Fromm, and others. She notes that she has tried to be objective in discussing that history but "being human, I must have blind spots" (p. v).

At Pembroke, in her class with Lindsay Damon Thompson, she was advised to think for herself, "not to take . . . [ideas] 'off the counter' as Damon had called it" (Capelle, 1993, p. 152). He promoted a skepticism about received ideas and, like other humanists of the era, rejected the pessimistic strain of European culture. He retained an earnest concern with morality and ethics, endorsing, as he once wrote, "belief in the worth of 'Good-deeds,' and . . . a historical survey of analysis is necessary for a thorough understanding" (Capelle, 1993, p. 153). The strength of this canon influenced her personality as well as her leadership style. It could be interpreted as diffidence. It is easy to be distracted by her modesty and thereby overlook her strengths (Harris (2017). From our 21st-century perch, we might want to mentor Thompson's approach to her talk: Don't be anxious and timid; don't appear to ask permission to speak about this history. Harris suggests, "who else could write such a lecture?" (p. 32). But Thompson is not there yet. It would take time for her to own her observations outright, and sadly, she does not have decades ahead of her. This is Thompson's story told in her voice, with all its strengths and limitations. We should not get stuck in the apparent hesitancy in her personality. There is much more to her than that surface reticence or seemingly docile cooperation.

Marylou Schimel Lionells, the former WAWI director, wondered, "Why didn't Clara Thompson wish to found a school in her own image as many have done in our field and why did she set up the Institute with a lay board?" In 1992, Lionells became the first woman to serve as Director following Thompson. She asked, "[W]hy did [Thompson] she urge graduates to leave rather than become acolytes?" Edgar Levenson put the question a little differently: "Why didn't Thompson create a following?" he mused, "that is how your name stays alive" (personal communication).

These questions touch on an aspect of Thompson's character that reappears throughout her life story—Thompson's unassumingness and her humility, her as she describes it, her compulsive modesty. She did not promote herself, and as for her ideas, she expected that they would be considered but not idealized. She did not fetishize theory. On the contrary, she encouraged a philosophical openness. One example of how that worked is given by Roanne Barnett (1989), who speaking of her father, Joseph Barnett, recalls how the senior Barnett was dissatisfied with his training at the Horney institute because of the demand for strict adherence to Horney's theories. He consulted Clara Thompson and she encouraged him to transfer to the WAWI. He studied there with Harry Bone, Erich Fromm, Rose Spiegel, and Meyer Maskin—presumably as his daughter opines, without the burden of the rigidity of specific theories or any one person.

In Her Own Image

Thompson did not want a school fashioned after her ideas. That would have run counter to her beliefs. She believed that independent thinkers would move the needle on what could be learned about human behavior. Time and again, she said it would benefit the field for people to develop their own thoughts. Founding an institute in her own image would go against both her humility and her belief in the benefits of cultivating free thinkers. Naming the institute after William Alanson White upheld a connection of psychoanalysis with psychiatry, her professional home base.

> In terms of the board of WAW, Thompson installed a diverse board of professionals that included a variety of people from business and law. She likely thought it wise for the Board to link the institute with the larger world, rather than with the more limited interests of psychoanalysts. She was aware of the institute as an enterprise, and she was determined for it to succeed. She may have thought that a board comprised of psychoanalysts could get bogged down in discussions driven by theoretical differences. Under her leadership she appointed the attorney, Abe Fortas, to a Board of Trustee position. He was very instrumental in disputes with the American Psychoanalytic Association. Fortas, a prominent Great Society liberal and adviser to Lyndon Johnson, was appointed to the Supreme Count but resigned under the cloud of scandal. He was an advocate of civil rights, social reform, and social justice. He saw similarities between lawyers and psychiatrists, noting that both groups focused on troubled individuals and "considered his meetings with clients as the occasions for transference" (Kalman, 1990, p. 178). Kenneth Eisold,[15] president of the WAW Board of Trustees in 2021, suggests that Thompson by insisting that "an institute is not a home" may have been trying to emphasize its role in the larger world. Fromm described Thompson as one of these rare persons who could take a leading role in the formation of an independent psychoanalytic group and continue to guide it. She was a thoroughly independent person, averse to rules and principles with which she did not agree; at the same time, she did not endow her own theoretical principles with a halo that would make her fight all others.
>
> (Fromm 1964, p. vi)

The years Thompson served as Director took an emotional toll added to the loss of many close colleagues and friends, including her partner Henry Major. Reflecting on those years, Ruth Moulton (1986) suggests that "although Thompson died of cancer, it might as well have been 'a broken heart,' such was her personal and professional disappointment in her last years" (p. 92).

In 1993–1994, WAW celebrated its 50th anniversary and memorialized their founders. Lionells (1995) comments that

> one participant wondered how this independent, yet shy woman could manage to maintain an atmosphere where two such powerful and contentious spirits as Harry Stack Sullivan and Erich Fromm could feel equally appreciated and comfortable.
>
> (Lionells, p. 63)

The truth is it came at a high cost. Perhaps she kept that hidden. Thompson had always been physically active, but fatigue plagued her in the last years. She gave up drinking and attempted to reduce physical stress but could not forestall the deterioration in her health. She remained at the helm of the Institute until her last days.

Notes

1 April 2, 1956, letter from Thompson to Fromm (housed in the Erich Fromm Archive, Tubingen).
2 Erich Fromm was also ostracized from the International Psychoanalytic Association (See The Exclusion of Erich Fromm from the IPA, Paul Roazen, 2001).
3 Perry explains there had been a growing sentiment "throughout the psychiatric community that would eventually define Sullivan as a radical and a somewhat dangerous professional friend; not all of his psychiatric colleagues agreed" but Perry explains, after his death he was "politically suspect as if he had been Karl Marx himself" (p. 326).
4 Letter dated March 11, 1956, Thompson to Fromm (housed in the Erich Fromm Archive, courtesy of Rainer Funk, Erich Fromm Archive, Tubingen).
5 Letter dated March 15, 1956, Fromm to Thompson (courtesy of Rainer Funk, Erich Fromm Archive, Tubingen).
6 Letter dated March 15, 1956, Fromm to Thompson, (courtesy of Rainer Funk, Erich Fromm Archive, Tubingen).
7 Letter dated April 3, 1956, Fromm to Thompson (courtesy of Rainer Funk, Erich Fromm Archive, Tubingen).
8 Vii Letter dated April 8, 1956, Thomposn to Fromm (housed in the Erich Fromm Archive, Tubingen).

9 He was also a crusader against same sex sexuality.

> No one knows the actual extent of homosexuality . . . Recently, I had a young homosexual who could pick up four partners just going from my office to the subway. What is the critical percentage for the presence of this brood? Is it a reversible trend? . . .. We owe our great civilization to the monogamous family . . .. Homosexuals have no vested interest in the future. And bisexuality is a homosexual compromise in which you can have your cake and your penny.
>
> (p. 218)

10 Letter dated April 8, 1956, Thompson to Fromm letter (housed in the Erich Fromm Archive, Tubingen).
11 Letter dated April 12, 1956, Fromm to Thompson (housed in the Erich Fromm Archive, Tubingen).
12 Letter dated May 4, 1956, Thompson to Fromm (housed in the Erich Fromm Archive, Tubingen).
13 Letter dated October 8, 1956, Thompson to Fromm (housed in the Erich Fromm Archive, Tubingen).
14 Letter dated November 24, 1956, Fromm dated Thompson to Fromm (housed in the Erich Fromm Archive, Tubingen).
15 Kenneth Eisold personal communication March 6, 2021.

References

Barnett, R. (1989). Joseph Barnett, MD, 1926–1988: In memoriam. *Contemporary Psychoanalysis, 25*, 663–666.

Bibring, E. (1950, May 18). Letter to Clara Thompson. The Oskar Diethelm Library, DeWitt Wallace Institute of Psychiatry: History, Policy, & the Arts, Weill Cornell Medical College. The Ralph Crowley Papers, Box 3, Fol. 1., New York, NY.

Capelle, E. L. (1993). Analyzing the "modern woman": Psychoanalytic debates about feminism, 1920–1950 (Unpublished doctoral dissertation). Columbia University.

Friedman, L. J. (2013). *The lives of Erich Fromm, Love's Prophet.* New York: Columbia University Press.

Fromm, E. (1956–1957). Letters to Clara Thompson. (March, 15, 1956, April 3, 1956, April 12, 1956.) Courtesy of Dr. Rainer Funk, Literary Estate of Erich Fromm, Erich Fromm Institute Tubingen.

Fromm, E. (1958, June 14). Freud, Friends, and Feuds: Scientism or Fanaticism? *The Saturday Review, 41*(14.6.), 11–13.

Fromm (1964). Forward. Erich Fromm, p. v–vi. In M. Green (Ed.), *Interpersonal psychoanalysis: The selected papers of Clara M. Thompson.* New York and London: Basic Books.

Frosch, J. (1991). The New York psychoanalytic civil wars. *Journal of the American Psychoanalytic Association, 39*, 1037–1064.

Green, M. R. (1964). Her life. p. 347–377 In M. R. Green (Ed.), *Interpersonal psychoanalysis: the selected papers of Clara M. Thompson*. New York: Basic Books.

Harris, A. (2017). Clara Thompson: What goes around . . . *Contemporary Psychoanalysis*, *3*(1), 32–36.

Kalman, L. (1990). *Abe Fortas: A biography*. New Haven, CT: Yale University Press.

Kardiner, A. (1978). The social distress syndrome of our time, part 2. *Journal of the American Academy of Psychoanalysis*, *6*(2), 215–230.

Kwawer, J. (2019). The interpersonal legacy of chestnut lodge. *Contemporary Psychoanalysis*, *55*(1–2), 86–98.

Landis, B., & Tauber, E. (Eds.). (1971). *In the name of life: Essays in honor of Erich Fromm*. New York: Holt, Rinehart and Winston.

Lionells, M. (1995). Clara M. Thompson (1893–1958), Some effects of the derogatory attitude toward female sexuality. Introduction. In D. Stern, C. Mann, S. Kantor, & G. Schlesinger (Eds.), *Pioneers of interpersonal psychoanalysis* (pp. 61–72). Hillside, NJ: The Analytic Press.

Moulton, R. (1969). My memories of being supervised. *Contemporary Psychoanalysis*, *5*(2), 151–157.

Moulton, R. (1975). Early papers on women: Horney to Thompson. *American Journal of Psychoanalysis*, *35*(3), 207–223.

Moulton, R. (1986). Clara Thompson, MD: Unassuming leader. In L. Dickstein & C. C. Nadelson (Eds.), *Women physicians in leadership roles* (p. 92). Washington, DC: American Psychiatric Press.

Perry. H. S. (1982). *Psychiatrist of America: The life of Harry Stack Sullivan*. Cambridge, MA: Belknap Press of Harvard University Press.

Spiegel, R. (1987). On receiving the distinguished service award. *Contemporary Psychoanalysis*, *23*, 2–5.

Thompson, C. (1938). *Introductory remarks*. Courtesy of WAWI Archives. William Alanson White Institute.

Thompson, C. (1942). Cultural pressures in the psychology of women. *Psychiatry*, *5*(3), 331–339.

Thompson, C. (1945) Transference as a Therapeutic Instrument, *Psychiatry, 8*, 273–278.

Thompson, C. (1950). *Psychoanalysis: Evolution and development*. New York: Hermitage.

Thompson, C. (1950, May 17). Letter to Edward Bibring. The Oskar Diethelm Library, DeWitt Wallace Institute of Psychiatry: History, policy, & the arts, Weill Cornell Medical College. The Ralph Crowley Papers, Box 3, Fol. 1., New York, NY.

Thompson, C. (1950, May 16). Letter to Edward Bibring. The Oskar Diethelm Library, DeWitt Wallace Institute of Psychiatry: History, Policy, & the Arts, Weill Cornell Medical College. The Ralph Crowley Papers, Box 3, Fol. 1., New York, NY.

Thompson, C. (1950, May 29). Letter to Edward Bibring. The Oskar Diethelm Library, DeWitt Wallace Institute of Psychiatry: History, policy, & the arts,

Weill Cornell Medical College. The Ralph Crowley Papers, Box 3, Fol. 1., New York, NY.

Thompson, C. (1956–1957). Letters to Erich Fromm. (March 11, 1956, April 2, 1956, April 8, 1956, May 4, 1956, October 8, 1956, November 24, 1956.) Housed in the Erich Fromm Archive, Courtesy of Rainer Funk, Erich Fromm Archive, Tubingen.

Thompson, C. (1958). A study of the emotional climate of psychoanalytic institutes. *Psychiatry, 21*(1), 45–51.

Thompson, C. (2017). The history of the William Alanson White Institute. *Contemporary Psychoanalysis, 53*(1), 7–28.

Chapter 7

Written Out of History

Death by Silence

> The minute she died; she was gone.
> (Personal communication, 2020, Edgar Levenson)

Despite her many accomplishments, Clara Thompson was quickly erased from psychoanalytic history. One would have expected the syllabi of our analytic training institutes to include the groundbreaking scholarly work of this pioneering leader, but it is absent. At my own institute New York University Postdoctoral Program in Psychotherapy and Psychoanalysis, as of this writing, there is no course on the work of Clara M. Thompson nor is there one at the training her Institute, the WAWI. As we contemplate her disappearance, there are some contributory factors and questions to consider. First and foremost is, Thompson's association with Ferenczi, which is critical in light of the decades-long ouster of his work from psychoanalysis. Brennan (2009) reviewing the contributions of the work of another of Ferenczi's unappreciated analysands, Izette de Forest, suggests,

> A pattern of disappearing persons seems to perpetuate itself in Ferenczi's legacy. Not only were Ferenczi and his ideas subject to repression after his death, but this process continues among his successors, though it may be viewed as the fragmentation and dissociation that occur as a result of trauma, which must then be slowly undone through a reliving such as the one we are collectively undertaking by gluing back together the lacerated soul bequeathed by Ferenczi to psychoanalysis.
> (p. 430)

Second, could Thompson's disappearance be the result of her career being shortened by death at the age of 65? Would ten or more years have made

DOI: 10.4324/9781003284840-8

a difference in establishing a legacy? Third, there was a paradigm shift in the culture of psychoanalysis that may be responsible for her disappearance. It was not long after her death that psychoanalysis became steeped in philosophy. But, Thompson was not a rigid person and understanding the impact of cultural shifts was her forte. Perhaps if she had lived, she would have evolved with the culture.

Then there is her "compulsive humility," was her humility detrimental to the continuation of her ideas? Her contemporaries, Harry Stack Sullivan, Karen Horney, and Erich Fromm, were not modest people; each promoted themselves and their ideas, and courted disciples thus leaving behind a recognizable legacy. Their behavior was more subtle perhaps than Freud who tried to secure his position by courting loyalty and bestowing rings to an inner circle of followers (Grosskurth, 1991).

Did her traumatic experience of physical abuse or, the speculated but unverified sexual abuse, contribute to her identified diffidence or detached manner—qualities that would not amass a following?

Why didn't Harry Stack Sullivan acknowledge Thompson's influence on his work in view of the long and productive association with her? Wolstein (1984) argues,

> In the "Conceptions," he [Sullivan] acknowledges three major predecessors to his thinking—Freud, Meyer, and White. Yet, we search those lectures in vain for a detailed, interwoven working-out of his intellectual and scientific relations to these three acknowledged figures. Nor, of course, do we find him making extensive, critical references to the contributions of those working along parallel lines in other perspectives, including the interpersonal humanism of the person with whom he most intimately worked, Thompson.
>
> (p. 212)

In her biography of Sullivan, Perry (1982) devotes a full chapter to their relationship, entitled, "Clara Thompson, Dear Friend and Colleague" (p. 201). Perry citing several other references notes Thompson's importance to Sullivan.

When Benjamin Wolstein was interviewed by Irwin Hirsch (2000), he explained his gratitude to Thompson:

> Why I hold Clara in such esteem is she wasn't afraid of knowing herself. She had great therapeutic courage. And, for reasons I never got

into with her, she was willing to go with me on it. For all I know, some patients did, still others didn't go there. But I did. I've come to this new mantra, "Wolstein's Law": Every therapist is unique, every patient is unique, every dyad is unique. The wider the range of capacity that a therapist has, or more exactly, capability, the greater the willingness to go into many different strange and secret places with patients. Such things make it possible for a therapist to work with a wider range of people beyond conscious and preconscious experience, in greater personal depth, beyond the borders of intimacy to the threshold of love.

(p. 187)

Wisely, Wolstein maintained:

To appreciate the core of Thompson's major contribution, we must, instead, look elsewhere. That is, to the impact of her direct experience and clinical psychoanalytic inquiry with her colleagues and students. She fostered, among those who closely followed her, a strong sense of fidelity to the actual clinical data, especially, in her personal view, when taking the analysis of transference and countertransference to what she considered its unanalyzable limits of involvement, with an open mind, however, to any new formulation that would recast the overly generalized aspects of the established metapsychologies built for interpreting the data. Most of all, as already suggested, she was concerned about reconstructing from a fresh point of view the instinctual-libidinal perspective of the earlier id and the later id-ego meta-psychologies with respect to the psychoanalysis of women. Essentially as a clinician and teacher, she made her influence most deeply felt in the life and work of many psychoanalysts at the Washington School of Psychiatry and at its New York Branch, including, the life and work of the subject of Perry's biographical study [Harry Stack Sullivan].

(Hirsch, p. 210)

Thompson's former analysand Erwin Singer, restated her ideas.

If the analytic process represents a series of situations in which all the patient's acts, be they commissions or omissions, reveal him . . . then exactly the same must be true for the analyst.

(Singer, 1977, p. 183)

But Singer referenced Fromm rather than Thompson:

> I am not talking about the analyst merely sharing with the patient events or facts of his life. . . . I am talking about a much more subtle process in which the patient, in exposing the structure and content of his concerns, simultaneously reveals what Fromm once called the person's private religion or the genuine hierarchy of values by which he lives no matter what fancy pretenses he may cherish or proffer. Similarly, the structure, focus and content of the analyst's response to the patient reveals the analyst's private religion, no matter what his pretense to himself and others.
>
> (p. 183)

Death by Association With Ferenczi

Silencing dissent has a deep history. In psychoanalysis it began with Freud. He repeatedly hurled personal attacks at those who disagreed with him; Ferenczi was immature, Jung puritanical, and Adler had an inferiority complex by dint of his small stature. Conceivably the most effective method used to silence critics was identified by Rachman (2018) as *Todschweigen*, or death by silence. It was practiced by Freud and utilized over generations (see Kurzweil, 2012; Menaker, 1989; Rachman, 1999, 2018). Poignantly, Esther Menaker recalls her class in Vienna when Ferenczi's death was announced, and no one spoke a word (Rachman, 2015). It was clear to her, we don't speak of Ferenczi, "they silenced him to death" (pp. 155–164). Kurzweil (2012) explains how that technique led to the disappearance of the work of psychoanalytic rebels from the 1930s and 1940s.

> Most of the participants in the quarrels of the 1940s are dead or retired from institutional politics. Active members tend not to know about this history, although their training has led them to practice what has been passed down from them.
>
> (p. 60)

Donnel Stern (2017) contextualizes the residue of that ghosted experience very well:

> I never knew Clara (I came along nearly 20 years after), but sometimes I feel that I must have known her, because she feels familiar to

me in a way that I am sure is also felt by many others who were trained long after her death.

(p. 4)

Michael Balint (1979) provides something else to consider:

> The historic event of the disagreement between Freud and Ferenczi acted as a trauma on the psychoanalytic world . . . the shock was highly disturbing and extremely painful. The first reaction to it was a frightened withdrawal.
>
> (p. 181)

In my interviews with contemporary psychoanalysts, I found few who had any substantive knowledge about Clara Thompson or her work. Some candidates in training at WAW knew little beyond her name, except that she was a founding member, and that a portrait of her hangs in the library. Kay (2014) who trained in the mid-west, discovered Clara Thompson as a central figure in New York's "fascinating history of political intrigue surrounding psychoanalysis." He notes,

> Her career was certainly colorful and I will assume that perhaps other readers, like me, know little of the intrigue or of her writing. Indeed, in neither my residency nor at the psychoanalytic institute, had I ever been assigned to read anything from her or about her. I can recall no teacher even mentioning her. Her absence in my education may reflect the provincialism of my teachers or my lack of initiative in reading beyond the assigned papers or both.
>
> (p. 1)

In an exchange of letters in the fall of 1957 (October 31, 1957, November 5, 1957, and November 12, 1957) housed in the Erich Fromm Archive, Tubingen., Fromm and Thompson discuss their outrage over Jones's allegations regarding Ferenczi's state of mind. "I thought of writing Jones," she says, "but he already has me labeled as deluded" (Thompson to Fromm letter November 5, 1957, housed in the Erich Fromm Archive, Tubingen). Silencing people by "diagnosing" them as mentally ill was a frequent strategy used to discredit. Fromm (1957) was shocked when he read Jones's book. He called it a "Stalinist type of re-writing history, whereby

Stalinists assassinate the character of opponents by calling them spies and traitors." (Fromm, 1958, p. 11) Rainer Funk pointed me to a work of Fromm's published remarks under the title "Psychoanalysis—Scientism or Fanaticism?" in *The Saturday Review*, New York, Vol. 41 (14.6.1958), pp. 11–13.55f., and included under the title *Freud, Friends, and Feuds*. Additionally important is Fromm's *The Dogma of Christ and Other Essays on Religion*, New York (Holt, Rinehart and Winston) 1963, pp. 93–102.

In Thompson's (1950) Introduction to the *Selected Papers of Sándor Ferenczi, Contributions to Psychoanalysis*, Volume I., she addresses in print the indictment by Jones against Ferenczi.

> Jones makes a statement which none of us who were there and saw Ferenczi frequently near the time of his death can understand— namely that he died insane with "maniacal and homicidal outbursts." The origin of this misrepresentation is a mystery. Balint, I and several others who saw him often in this period saw no evidence of it. Not only is it implied that he was insane at the time of his death, but also that his psychosis had been developing for several years. In other words, all his last work, with especial emphasis on his paper *Confusion of Tongues*, found in Volume III of the *Selected Papers of Sándor Ferenczi*, are supposedly the products of a disordered mind. And yet what Ferenczi said in that paper is current analytic practice with many analysts today. It seems that his crime was that he was twenty years ahead of his time and did not agree with his leader.
>
> (Thompson, 1950, *Introduction*, Contributions to Psychoanalysis)

Her published denial of Jones's accusations may very well factor in why her work like Ferenczi's disappeared from the literature.

A Paradigm Shift

Edgar Levenson offers another framework in which to consider Thompson's erasure. While Thompson was a politically important person at the WAW institute, as he recalls it, "the minute she died, she was gone" (E. Levenson, January, 2020, personal communication). He suggests her disappearance was not so much about her but coincident with a paradigm shift in the psychoanalytic culture, particularly at William Alanson White (WAWI). He referred to the American physicist and philosopher, Thomas Kuhn (1962), who in *The Structure of Scientific Revolutions*, introduced the concept of "paradigm shift." Levenson suggests that psychoanalysts not only changed the way they thought about their work, and he added, the field itself was transformed under the influence of the women's movement.

The shift was an imperceptible incremental shift—to a more abstract discourse grounded in philosophy and away from Thompson's plainspoken language and practical theorizing. For example, analysts gravitated toward the more complex existentialism of Binswanger (May et al., 1958, p. 194). Levenson explains, "We thought philosophical thinking would give the institute legitimacy, respectability." Reflecting on the situation, he submits that for someone to persist in the psychoanalytic literature, they need the following: "You need a group of disciples." Thompson never cultivated disciples; on the contrary, she promoted independence.

Levenson (1972) was prescient in addressing paradigm shifts. He cited Marshall McLuhan and Buckminster Fuller's observations on technology and the wisdom of "the tool makes man as much as man makes the tool" (p. 48).

Thompson's analysand, Benjamin Wolstein (1962), argued,

> We are not the hollow generation that grew up in the psychological wastelands of thirty and forty years ago, not the lost generation of the twenties or the searching one of the thirties. Not only are we faced with new problems that demand specifically new resolutions, we are even compelled to create new ways to deal with the older ones. For our problems are no simple recurrence of theirs, and our opportunities are not confined to theirs. Those who reached intellectual maturity then are now looking for salvation in existentialism and mysticism. But they no longer speak to a generation that is hopelessly lost in the pleasure of each minute sensation: an experience, to be good, does not have to be good to the last drop.
>
> (p. 123)

Thompson's sense of independence led to what Levenson perceived as "an absence of being deeply embedded in theoretical systems." Her students took divergent paths. Levenson, one of the most distinguished thinkers in the past decades, introduced general systems theory and an interest in language into the analytic literature. In *Language and Healing* (Levenson, 1979), he took a giant step away from the practical, plainspoken style of Clara Thompson:

> Every psychoanalyst dreads that moment when some well-meaning naif corners him at a cocktail party and asks what it is we really do

with patients and we are obliged to answer, lamely, "Well, we talk with them." It seems a sorry virtuosity, this being masters of the commonplace. After all, everyone knows how to talk. Yet, as I shall elaborate, from a structural linguistic perspective on psychoanalytic process, there are extremely subtle and intricate ramifications to this most ordinary and unselfconscious function.

(p. 271)

Levenson closes his essay suggesting something to which Thompson would conceivably agree:

> The psychoanalyst—he who talks with his patients—then, is the person who is trying to understand and clarify an ordinary process, really most naturally performed without thinking too much about it. Cloaked in structuralist trappings, the inquiry has tones of grandeur. As Roland Barthes put it, "Once again the exploration of language, conducted by linguistics, psychoanalysis, and literature, corresponds to the exploration of the cosmos" (Barthes, 1970, p. 144). But, put in a humbler metaphor, we are perhaps like the centipede trying to figure out how we manage to put one foot in front of the other without falling on our faces in the process.
>
> (p. 281)

As Levenson reached for grand ideas, he was humbled by the process.

These examples offer just one way to understand Thompson's disappearance from the analytic literature—a cultural paradigm shift that left her behind.

Levenson continued what Thompson began, refined it, and elaborated it along the way. As he said,

> When I was in supervision with Clara Thompson, she used to say that if you started with a patient, and after the first week you found yourself thinking in terms of diagnosis, look to your countertransference. The idea being that the uneasier you became the more you began to diagnose, abstract, generalize, and so forth so.
>
> (Levenson, E. A., Hirsch, I., & Iannuzzi, V. (2005), p. 595)

His well-known quote, "[O]ne cannot *not* interact, one cannot *not* influence" (Levenson, 2009, p. 172), is legendary. For Levenson, language with its nuances of irony, sarcasm, humor, its, "(tonal, prosody) is the major instrument of mystification. He explained,

> Mystification and its concurrent anxiety operate most strongly in early life events, but current events reiterate the earlier patterning. It is not that the patient is wrong about the present, but the affect and, more important, the sense of semiotic confusion and impotence resonate powerfully with earlier experience. The patient is not wrong in perceptions, but the affect and sense of helplessness surely are.

It is not only speech but nonverbal nuances.

> I have elaborated on the body-mind link and on this very possibility— that learning may be first bodily, first imitative, mimetic, and *then* cerebral (Levenson, 1998). This idea suggests the interesting possibility that psychoanalytic insight may be first experienced and *then* formulated; that the direction of learning may be, not from the head to the body, but quite the opposite—a matter of what is said about what is experienced.
>
> (pp. 172–173)

This quote brings to my mind Donnel Stern's (1983) concept of unformulated experience suggesting to me that Thompson's impact made its way to Stern. As for Levenson (2009), language was understood as "less about communication of information than about deception and control— power" (p. 173). His words reflect those of Thompson, Sullivan, Horney, and Fromm. Foehl (2008) considers Levenson, "the best-known theorist of interpersonal psychoanalysis."

Thompson's clinical theories reverberate too in the work of Irwin Hoffman's (2006) dialectical-constructivist perspective. No doubt she would agree with some of his assertions concerning a set of myths about,

> the denial of the patient's agency (i.e. the **myth** that the patient is not a free agent); the denial of the patient's and the analyst's interpersonal influence (i.e. the **myth** that the patient and the analyst are largely unaffected by each other's interpersonal attitudes and actions); and the denial of the patient's share of responsibility for co-constructing the analytic relationship (i.e. the **myth** that the patient does not

share responsibility with the analyst for the quality of the analytic relationship).

(p. 44)

Compulsive Modesty

What about Thompson's personality can explain what happened? Her essays lean toward selflessness, as she minimizes her offerings. She tried to explain away her shyness by referring to herself as a "silent Swede," a nod to her distant Scandinavian background (Moulton, 1975). Spiegel (1987) observed how at times she compensated for her discomfort when lecturing by "being a little rebelliously witty and cheery" (p. 2). Edgar Levenson and Erwin Singer, who for two years shared a supervision hour with Thompson, experienced the "silent Swede." Levenson recalls that she was silent during most of the hour. After presenting their cases to Thompson, he and Singer met for coffee and wondered if they had done well. As their patients improved, they found themselves more confident in their work, suggesting that Thompson's methods were subtle but effective. Levenson finds that his thinking was highly influenced by Thompson. He recalled a diffident quality to her character and wondered if that contributed to the minimization of her legacy. (2020, personal communication).

Levenson (2002) Speaking of his early years at WAWI and his supervision with Thompson Levenson points to the importance of creative collaboration between the patient and analyst.

> I believe that Thompson, older and more imbedded in classical training than Moulton, had more interest in the associative play, the stream of consciousness.[3] Thompson said to me that she'd given up free association, not because she didn't find it uniquely valuable, but because most patients couldn't do it—"They just nattered on!" She also told me, with wry regret, that candidates didn't "seem to believe anymore in the unconscious." Moulton was much closer to Sullivan and Fromm-Reichman in her belief that behind the world of fantasy and phantasmagoria was a mystified reality, rendered incomprehensible and chaotic by the patient's unendurable anxiety. The play of imagination was part of the disease, not the cure.
>
> (2002, p. 280)

Thompson encouraged her students to find their own analytic voice rather than echoing hers—an admirable approach but not one that would create a "brand." This contrasted with Karen Horney, who was self-promoting. Rubins (1978) notes that in one two-year period, "at least five new-born baby daughters of candidates' wives were named after Karen" (p. 259).

Surely, her reserved character and what she refers to as her "compulsive modesty" were remnants of her deeply internalized Free Will Baptist values that taught her to put others before herself. Did that experience create a detached manner? Shapiro (1993) noted her detachment as suggestive of the sequelae of traumatic sexual abuse—that interpretation is based on the notation from Ferenczi's diary, a plausible misattribution that baffles us rather than informs.[1] Regardless, she suffered childhood trauma at the hand of a cold, critical, and abusive mother. Her repeated confusion in her interview with Kurt Eissler over whether Ferenczi's paper, *Confusion of Tongues*, was ever published promotes the speculation that this was a manifestation of dissociation.[2] We have also heard her state clearly that she knew the paper was published and what it concerned.

Erich Fromm knew Thompson well—as an analysand, a colleague, and a friend, giving him a complex understanding of her character. He describes her as, "a person who did not endow her own theoretical principles with a halo that would make her fight all others" (in Green, (1964) p. vi). In other words, she did not set herself up as an authority, nor did she demand loyalty or conformity to her ideas. In fact, she renounced all forms of authoritarianism and "acted according to her convictions" (p. vi). She never intimidated others; she was loyal and possessed integrity and common sense; she was also warm and nurturant.

Moulton (1975) remarks that Thompson's contributions were partly overlooked because they often seemed like "common sense," "like something we always knew but, one should add, paid little attention to" (p. 217). These glowing accounts sit alongside of the fact that she could at times grow silent and seem detached.

We need to be vigilant about holding in higher esteem those who weave ideas about human experiences into a complicated jargon, while diminishing those who use a language that is clear and straightforward, labeling it somehow less intellectual. This holdover was in part from an early insecurity that used scientific language to impress and attain legitimacy. Can we now say it has lost its usefulness?

Waugaman (2016) points out that Thompson never sought out the limelight:

> Her modest tendency to mediate between conflicting analytic factions did not bring her into the limelight (Waugaman, 2014). She achieves an enviable balance in her opinions, whereas analysts who advocate more extreme positions may draw greater attention to their work.
>
> (p. 13)

Waugaman also observes how authors quote Thompson second hand without citing her directly.

The Long Reach of Sexism

Thompson's erasure can also be understood the result of sexism exacerbated following the second World War. Rose Spiegel (1997), one of the first students to graduate from the new WAW Institute, recalls when she began training in the early 1940s, "there just weren't any males, not till the war was well on its way out" (p. 186). This made room for Thompson, who Spiegel saw as a "powerful force"—by powerful, she explains, "almost like an engine" (p. 2). According to Spiegel

> the post-Depression and War years of the 1940's were the Great Divide for psychoanalysis and for societal changes. When I began with Clara in 1942, I was impressed with the very alive professional role of women psychoanalysts—there were Karen Horney, Clara Thompson, Janet Rioch, Frieda Fromm-Reichmann. Clara was both sensitive and sturdy, pragmatic in the best sense and romantic. In fact, if not in label, she was an early feminist and saw the strength in women, and was very sensitive to and caring for men. My attraction to Clara had begun with the warmth of her voice over the phone and was re-enforced by the presence of Masha, her cat. Clara and I shared an abiding interest in felines.
>
> (p. 2)

Women in the 1950s in America, and around the world, were marginalized, exploited, patronized, subjected to violence, and oppressed within a male-dominated culture. Their aspirations were minimized or discounted entirely. Betty Friedan's, *The Feminine Mystique* (1963) named the malaise women felt as, "The problem that has no name." The women Friedan interviewed were privileged white women who described their isolation and unhappiness; they experienced a generalized feeling of wanting more out of life.

A more recent example of the impact of sexism is heard in a statement by John Kelly, the White House chief of staff who opined how when he was growing up, "women were sacred, looked upon with great honor." The reporter Eric Zorn (2017), with the byline, *Women Were Marginalized in the 1950s, Not Consecrated*, offered a cultural artifact from the era that exemplifies the sexism that dominated American society in the 1950s. He offers,

> A 1952 magazine ad for Chase & Sanborn coffee, for instance, shows a man preparing to spank a woman whom he's thrown across his lap. "If your husband ever finds out you're not 'store testing' for fresher coffee . . ." says the ad copy, "woe be unto you."
>
>   (Chicago Tribune, Eric Zorn, 10/20/17)

This advertisement is a form of "hostile sexism" that was pervasive in the culture that Clara Thompson encountered daily. As a professional, unmarried woman, she was always suspected of not being a real woman. For women in the 1950s, the only legitimate goal sanctioned by society was the pursuit of a man (Friedan, 1963). In their research, psychologists Peter Glick and Susan Fisk (1996) categorized two dimensions of sexism. They coined the terms "hostile sexism" and "benevolent sexism." The statement by White House Chief of Staff John Kelly is a form of "benevolent sexism" that follows a "set of stereotypical beliefs toward women that express a sense of protective paternalism and chivalry. These beliefs rely upon traditional gender roles to place women on pedestals" (Glick & Fisk, 1996, p. 491). Both forms of sexism were and still are widespread.

Cosmopolitan Interview

Cosmopolitan, with a circulation of over one million readers, was a leading magazine that combined a quasi-sophisticated mix of pop culture, prose, and romance. The March 1955 issue contains an interview with Clara Thompson. It has a photo of the actress Eva Marie Saint on the cover. The charmingly straightforward interview conducted by the Hollywood writer, and biographer, Maurice Zolotow, contains a few surprises.

Thompson demonstrates her ability to communicate clearly to and appeal to a wide-ranging audience. Her appearance in this widely circulated magazine does not prevent or forestall her fading from history.

Q. Dr. Thompson, I'm going to put to you the questions I think the readers of COSMOPOLITAN would like to ask you if they were privileged to sit here with you.

To begin with, I think you'll agree with me that the average person is still in the dark as to just what people in your branch of the medical profession do.

A. Well, psychiatry is the treatment of diseases—disturbances of human functioning—but they're not organic or bodily diseases they're diseases produced by something's going wrong in a person's life situation . . .

Q. When do you think a person ought to consult a psychoanalyst?

A. There are two types of people at the extreme of human difficulties . . . the person who is so disturbed and full of anxiety he will not respond to easily to being reshaped except by deep therapy. It might be somebody with melancholia or depressions so bad he is close to suicide. That is one sort of patient who could be helped by psychoanalysis at the other extreme is the person who is what I call a "going concern."

Q. By a "going concern," I take it you mean somebody who is holding down a job, who, though he may feel frustrated at the job or unhappy with his children or spouse at least has some kind of home life?

A. That's right. An increasing number of people who come for analysis belong in this group.

The interviewer is interested in knowing if an individual can decide whether they need an analysis. Thompson answers in the affirmative and explains that it is best if the person decides they *want* psychoanalysis, "in order to live more fully creatively," rather than that they need it. She explains that those most in need often are pushed into analysis, but it is impossible to analyze someone against their will.

Q. In addition to feelings of misery or unhappiness that may make a person want analysis—are there definite physical symptoms that indicate the need for analysis? I have in mind what we call psychosomatic diseases and such conditions as high blood pressure, ulcers, and migraine.

A. No. In itself, no one of these diseases would indicate the need for treatment. We do know, however, that emotions—suppressed hostility, frustration, rage—can adversely affect breathing, blood circulation and secretions in the stomach. But the patient with organic symptoms should consult their doctor first before considering undergoing psychoanalysis.

The interviewer questions Thompson about the expressions "mental hygiene" and "mental illness." Thompson responds, explaining that the word "mental" is a hangover from old-fashioned thinking. Contemporary psychiatrists deal with "the whole body under emotional stress." The next question is about the capacity to determine who needs treatment and if there is a feeling that everyone can use a "good analysis."

A. Theoretically, everyone would benefit by psychoanalysis. But you have to consider several things. First, does the patient really want it after you have explained it to him? Secondly, is he open minded? Is he capable of change? In other words, one has to consider how rigid he is. The rigid person is not a good analysis risk.

Q. By rigid you mean . . . ?

A. Well, there are some men and women who cannot do anything out of their set routine—they just cannot do it. They're the kind of persons you can set your clock by, as the saying goes. Things have got to go the way they have always gone; they have to believe what they have always believed. Another thing you have to consider—in sizing up a person as a prospect for analysis—is the age of the person not so much in terms of his chronological age but in terms of his flexibility his potential development. 96

Q. Do you feel that some people lose the ability to grow and change at thirty and others can still grow and change at sixty?

A. In some cases, yes, and in other cases it isn't just that they have lost the ability to change, but some people have succeeded in getting themselves into situations they cannot get out of. For instance, a woman who all her life has been too neurotic to accept herself as a woman and has been unable to get married comes for analysis at fifty. She probably can't get married even if you help her with her problem—it might be shyness for instance. On the other hand, if the analysis is successful, the person will find vital, constructive substitutes, goals of life, ways to express herself, even if it is too late to be married. (Zolotow, 1955, pp. 64–65) 302

Wait, what? "A woman who all her life has been too neurotic to accept herself as a woman"? Is this our pioneering feminist? What happened to the cultural analysis she provided in *"The Role of Women in This Culture"* (1941) and the historical analysis she provided in *"Cultural Pressures in the Psychology of Women"* (1942)? Did Thompson believe that the best this 50-year-old woman who enters analytic treatment can hope for is to find constructive substitutes for love and partnership? Rather, does she mean that women should not focus so much on marriage, that there are other important and satisfying goals in life?

Let's step back and look at this issue of *Cosmopolitan* with a wider lens. It is 1955. The actress Eva Marie Saint has just received accolades for her performance in the award-winning film *On the Waterfront*, earning her an academy award for her performance. In Saint's interview, she is pregnant and describes how she is "looking forward eagerly to her baby" (Gehman, 1955, p. 63), which will be born the following month. "The pregnancy," she explains, "has not handicapped her in TV: considerate directors have shot her from the waist up" (p. 63). She does not believe that having a child will hamper her in any way. "If anything, the career will bow to the child" (p. 63), she says. Some measure of the relative importance she places on each of these parts of her life may be gleaned from how she describes finding out she was pregnant. She explains, she went to her friendly neighborhood druggist for a test; on the day the result was due, she was in the store bright and early. " 'Mrs. Hayden, congratulations,' says the druggist. 'You mean—?' 'I mean,' he said. 'The reviews of *Waterfront* were great.' Her smile vanished. She looked crestfallen. 'Oh,' she said. 'that'" (p. 63). Despite her accomplished career, motherhood was what is most important. Psychoanalytic theories in the 1950s would concur underscoring biology and women's nature. But as Thompson noted, it was cultural pressures that lead women to feel their destiny is motherhood.

Returning to the interview, Zolotow (1955) asks a set of questions including the frequency and length of sessions. Thompson explains that a classic analyst might feel four times a week is necessary, but she thinks that the number of visits a week does not determine whether a treatment is psychoanalytic. It is more the type of therapy being conducted. Sessions she explains are usually 45–50 minutes long. The cost of analysis is discussed, and she points out that several institutes offer low-cost services at about $15 an hour and that lying on a couch is not necessary. She describes how that was Freud's original method but only the classical school still sees it that way. The interviewer then turns to what happens during the session. Who talks? Is it the patient or does the analyst talk too? Thompson describes how listening is the most critical part of the analytic situation because the analyst is trying to find out if the patient is doing with or to the analyst what he does with others "as well as understand the obvious surface meaning of what he is saying to him." The analyst can sometimes "see beneath the words of the patient, he has to bring this all together and point out things to the patient the patient isn't aware of himself." Thompson explains that

> there might be emotions present, too. There might be joy. There might be grief. In short, anything can happen when one talks to a friend one trusts; what two people who feel close to each other and are trying to understand each other might be doing. Except that in this situation, the analyst is not concerned with talking about himself or his difficulties. He is there to help the patient for the patient's sake.

The interviewer wonders how a simple exchange can accomplish improvement in the patient. She responds, "[I]t's more than "getting something off your chest" though "catharsis helps." More important, or fully as important, is learning about the things you do with people, which create difficulties in human relations. The interviewer gives an example of a situation where a man loses job after job because he insults people, gets into fights basically, and can't get along with others. He seeks help from an analyst and learns that this fighting with others "is an expression of a neurotic hostility which traces back to his early relations with his father. As soon as the patient knows this, will he stop getting into arguments?" Thompson explains that the analytic process is much more complicated.

A. The first step is to realize it may take a long time for a patient to realize how he is behaving and what he is really doing in his relations with people. Realizing this is what Sullivan called the big milestone in psychotherapy. It takes a long time to reach this milestone. The second

step is to see oneself doing it in hundreds of situations. The patient
during his visits reports what he has been doing since the previous session and what he is doing to destroy himself becomes pretty obvious
to the patient. But he still doesn't automatically change. There comes a
time however, when he begins to have an emotional awareness before
each time he is about to fight with somebody over something trivial.
It's something he feels, not something he thinks. A new element enters
in. He has a completely new human experience. And then someday he
does not fight. His personality finds a better way of integrating with
people. For the analysts this turning point of his patient is probably the
most spiritually rewarding experience the analysts can have.

Thompson's answer is poignant. It is interesting that she uses the word
"spiritually" rewarding rather than "emotionally" rewarding. Is this a
holdover from her early religious training?

Next, the interviewer wants to know if the patient must tell the analyst
everything. She answers, in the affirmative and explains,

[N]obody tells everything ever but that is the aim . . . in spite of everything, people censor their thoughts before speaking and it takes a
long time in any analysis for one to reach a point where he is capable
of complete frankness.

Q. What happens when a patient holds something back?

A. It just wastes time, period. It holds up the whole process of cure. Sometimes the patient unconsciously holds something back. Sometimes he
does this without realizing it. Sometimes it is deliberate.

Q. You have mentioned anxiety. What is anxiety?

A. Anxiety is a very unpleasant bodily sensation accompanied by sweat-
ing, rapid heartbeat, weakness in the knees, faulty breathing—as
though one has been threatened very badly. Of course, there are vary-
ing degrees of anxiety. You feel afraid but often you do not know what
it is you fear.

Q. Are the defensive things people do in their relations with other people—like the man who picks arguments with everybody—ways of
handling anxiety, defense mechanisms for keeping anxiety out of your
mind?

A. Usually, yes. It's the way you protect yourself from the unpleasant sensation of anxiety by doing something about it and that's called a defense. Often the things a person has become accustomed to doing as a way of checking his anxiety are self-destructive.

Thompson's replies offer the reader a straightforward understanding of the process of psychoanalysis with answers that are unencumbered with jargon. The interview ends with a question about children.

Q. Do you have any suggestions for parents of young children as to how to handle their children in such ways as to prevent their children from being neurotic in later life?

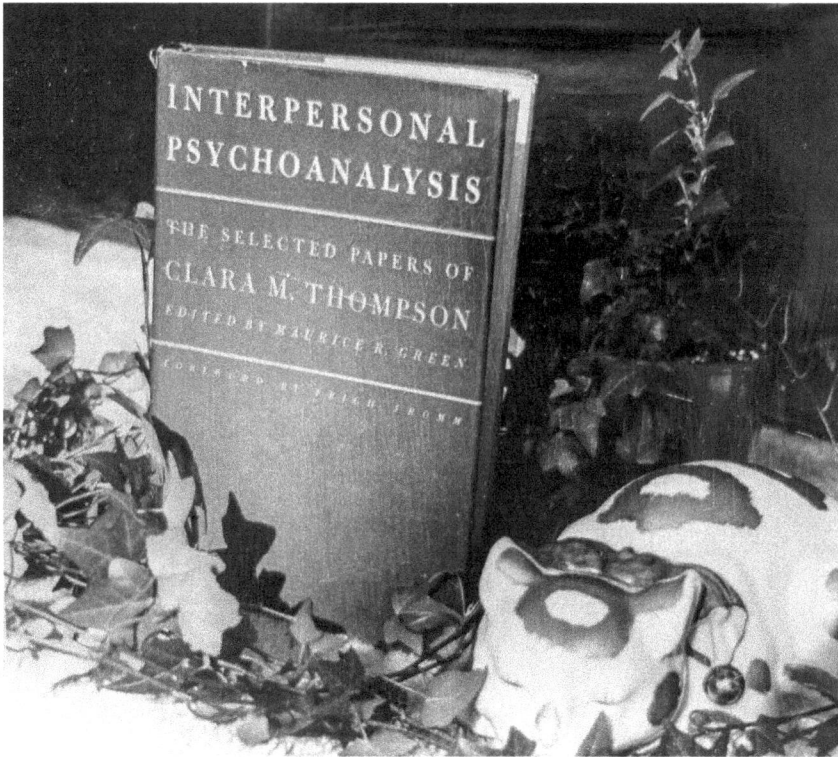

Figure 7.1 Interpersonal Psychoanalysis: The Selected Papers of Clara Thompson. Reprinted with permission, © William Alanson White Institute.

Thompson. The most important thing is for parents to love their children. The next most important thing is, failing love, to avoid being a hypocrite. This is very confusing to a child to have you pretend to be calm when you are furious inside. Being honest with a child even when

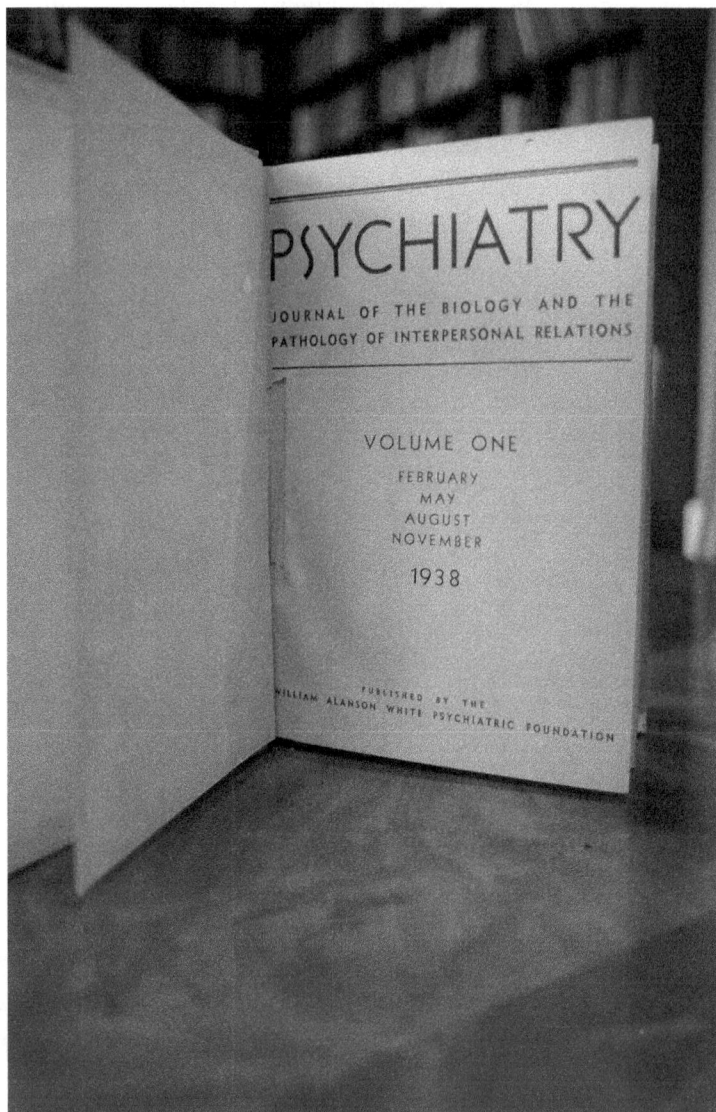

Figure 7.2 Psychiatry: Journal of the Biology and the Pathology of Interpersonal Relations. Volume 1, 1938. Image taken by the author.

you must show him your boredom or anger is better than faking some emotions you don't feel or striking some attitude you feel should be struck in the situation. But there is no substitute for genuine mother and father affection in making healthy human beings. (p. 69)

Thompson's answers go to the heart of being human, our need for love, and our need for honesty. She holds the audience's attention in a relaxed and informed tone. Today she would have a podcast or she might be given a talk show to host.

This *Cosmopolitan* interview, in its entirety, is archived in National Institute of Health (NIH) as part of an *Introductory Reading List on Mental Health* published by the US Department of Health, Education and Welfare.[3] Sometime over the following decade, her name would slowly be written out of history. The neglect of her legacy cannot become a norm we take for granted, but claiming her legacy requires that to paraphrase a title of an Adrienne Rich poem, we resist amnesia.

Notes

1 See chapter four in *Clara M. Thompson's Early Years and Professional Awakening: An American Psychoanalyst (1893–1933)*, Routledge Press.
2 Clara Thompson was identified as patient Dm. in Ferenczi's Clinical Diary. See *Clara M. Thompson's Early Years and Professional Awakening: An American Psychoanalyst (1893–1933)* for a full discussion.
3 Introductory Readings in Mental Health, March 1955, ref. guide, 3. Reprinted July 1959.

References

Balint, M. (1979). *The basic fault: Therapeutic aspects of regression*. New York: Brunner.
Barthes, R. (1970), in *The Structuralist Controversy*, R. Macksey and E. Donato, Eds., Johns Hopkins Press, Baltimore, p. 136.
Brennan, B. W. (2009). Ferenczi's forgotten messenger: The life and work of Izette de Forest. *American Imago*, 66(4), 427–455.
Foehl, J. (2008). Follow the Fox: Edgar A. Levenson's pursuit of psychoanalytic process. *The Psychoanalytic Quarterly*, 77(4), 1231–1268.
Friedan, B. (1963). *The feminine mystique*. New York: W. W. Norton & Company.
Fromm, E. (1957). Letters to Clara Thompson.
Fromm, E. (1958, June 14). Scientism or Fanaticism? *Saturday Review*, 41, 11–13.
Fromm, E. (1963). *The dogma of Christ and other essays on religion* (pp. 93–102). New York: Holt, Rinehart and Winston.

Fromm, E. (1964). Foreword. In M. R. Green (Ed.), *Interpersonal psychoanalysis: The selected papers of Clara M. Thompson* (pp. v–vi). New York: Basic Books.

Hirsch, I. (2000). Interview with Benjamin Wolstein. *Contemporary Psychoanalysis, 36*(2), 187–232.

Hoffman, I. Z. (2006). The myths of free association and the potentials of the analytic relationship. *International Journal of Psychoanalysis, 87*(1), 43–61.

Gehman, R. (1955, March). Eva Marie Saint—A new kind of star. *Cosmopolitan, 138*, pp. 58–63.

Glick, P., & Fisk, S. (1996). The ambivalent sexism inventory: Differentiating hostile and benevolent sexism. *Journal of Personality and Social Psychology, 70*(3), 491–512.

Grosskurth, P. (1991). *The secret ring: Freud's inner circle and the politics of psychoanalysis*. New York: Addison-Wesley and Addison Wesley Longman.

Kay, J. (2014). Commentary on Clara Thompson's transference as a therapeutic instrument: Foreseeing the real relaionship. *Psychiatry, 77*(1), 1–7.

Kuhn, T. (1962). *The structure of scientific revolutions*. Chicago IL: University of Chicago Press.

Kurzweil, E. (2012). Ferenczi in context. In J. Szekacs-Weisz & T. Keve (Eds.), *Ferenczi and his world: Rekindling the spirit of the Budapest school* (pp. 55–68). London: Routledge.

Levenson, E. A. (1972). *The fallacy of understanding*. New York: Basic Books.

Levenson, E. A. (1979). Language and healing. *Journal of the American Academy of Psychoanalysis, 7*(2), 271–282.

Levenson, E. A. (1998). Awareness, insight and learning. *Contemporary Psychoanalysis, 34*, 239–249.

Levenson, E. A. (2002). And the last shall be first: Some observations on the evolution of interpersonal psychoanalysis. *Contemporary Psychoanalysis, 38*(2), 277–285.

Levenson, E. A. (2005). Response to the commentaries. *Contemporary Psychoanalysis, 41*(4), 749–750.

Levenson, E. A. (2009). The enigma of the transference. *Contemporary Psychoanalysis, 45*(2), 163–178.

Levenson, E. A., Hirsch, I., & Iannuzzi, V. (2005). Interview with Edgar A. Levenson January 24, 2004. *Contemp. Psychoanal. 41*(4), 593–644.

May, R. E., Angel, E. E., & Ellenberger, H. F. (1958). *Existence: A new dimension in psychiatry and psychology*. New York: Basic Books.

Menaker, E. (1989). *Appointment in Vienna: An American psychoanalyst recalls her student days in pre-war Austria*. New York: St. Martin's Press.

Moulton, R. (1975). Early papers on women: Horney to Thompson. *American Journal of Psychoanalysis, 35*(3), 207–223.

Perry, H. S. (1982). *Psychiatrist of America*. Cambridge, MA: The Belknap Press of Harvard University Press.

Rachman, A. W. (1999). Todschweigen (Death by silence): The traditional practice of silencing dissidence in psychoanalysis. In R. Prince (Ed.), *Is psychoanalysis dead: Murder? suicide? or rumor greatly exaggerated?* (pp. 155–164). New York: Jason Aronson.

Rachman, A. W. (2015). Elizabeth Severn: Sándor Ferenczi's analysand and collaborator in the study of treatment of trauma. In A. Harris & S. Kuchuck (Eds.), *The legacy of Sándor Ferenczi: From ghost to ancestor*, 220. New York: Routledge Press.

Rachman, A. W. (2018). *Elizabeth Severn: The "evil genius" of psychoanalysis*. London: Routledge.

Rubins, J. L. (1978). *Karen Horney: Gentle rebel of psychoanalysis*. New York: The Dial Press.

Shapiro, S. A. (1993). Clara Thompson: Ferenczi's messenger with half a message. In L. Aron & A. Harris (Eds.), *The legacy of Sándor Ferenczi* (pp. 159–174). Hillsdale, NJ: The Analytic Press.

Singer, E. (1977). *The fiction of analytic anonymity* in K. Frank (Ed.) The Human Dimension in Psychoanalytic Practice. p. 181–192. Grune & Stratton, New York.

Spiegel, R. (1987). On receiving the distinguished service award. *Contemporary Psychoanalysis*, *23*(1), 2–5.

Spiegel, R. (1997). Reminiscences. *Contemporary Psychoanalysis*, *33*, 185–187.

Stern, D. (1983). Unformulated experience: From Familiar chaos to creative disorder. *Contemporary Psychoanalysis*, *19*, 71–99.

Stern, D. (2017). Interpersonal psychoanalysis: History and current status. *Contemporary Psychoanalysis*, *53*(1), 69–94.

Thompson, C. (1941). The role of women in this culture. *Psychiatry*, *4*(1), 1–8.

Thompson, C. (1942). Cultural pressures in the psychology of women. *Psychiatry*, *5*(3), 331–339.

Thompson, C. (1950). Introduction. In *The selected papers of Sándor Ferenczi, sex in psychoanalysis* (Vol. 1). New York: Basic Books.

Waugaman, R.M. (2014). "Remembering Sullivan's Psychoanalyst: Commentary on Clara Thompson's Transference as a Therapeutic Instrument." *Psychiatry 77*, 25–29.

Waugaman, R. M. (2016). Further notes on choosing an analyst. *Psychiatry*, *79*(1), 13–18.

Wolstein, B. (1962). On the psychological absurdity of existential analysis. *Psychoanalytic Review*, *49*(3), 117–124.

Wolstein, B. (1984). The interpersonal perspective of the American School. *Contemporary Psychoanalysis*, *20*, 204–223.

Zolotow, M. (1955, March). What you should know about psychiatry. *Cosmopolitan*, *138*, 64–69, US Department of Health, Education, and Welfare (NIH), reference guide 3.

Zorn, E. (2017). *Women were marginalized in the 1950s, not consecrated*. Chicago, IL: Chicago Tribune.

Chapter 8

The Legacy of Clara Mabel Thompson and On Touching the Future

Mortality

During the summer of 1956, Clara Thompson exhibited signs of illness. Green (1964) recalls during a visit to Provincetown, her "quieter than usual" demeanor, "although she was as warm and responsive as always, but there seemed to be a tired edge to her manner." Thompson brushed off her fatigue, attributing it to an "intestinal flu" (p. 374). When she returned to New York, her internist referred her to a surgeon. In October, the month of her 63rd birthday, a malignant polyp was removed, and a large bowel resection was performed. Thompson's doctors did not have access to today's diagnostic or therapeutic modalities of radiologic scans and chemotherapy. Instead, her doctors prescribed alcohol avoidance and a high protein diet. Her doctors were optimistic, and Thompson seems to have shared their optimism adjusting her diet and eliminating alcohol.

Green (1964a) recalls that during her hospitalization, she received many gifts, notes, and flowers and that she wanted to thank each person. To that end, she published a note in the fall issue of the WAW Newsletter thanking everyone.

Shortly after her discharge, she learned that a close friend too had undergone surgery for cancer and was now depressed. She phoned the friend with an invitation to come visit, but the friend declined. "An hour later her friend's doorbell rang, and Clara came in and sat down, telling her about the severe depression she used to have herself" (Green, p. 375).

Green (1964a) recalls,

> Clara either pretended or was persuaded not to know that a malignancy had been discovered in her colon. The story given out, and to all appearances accepted by her, was that an ordinary polyp was excised

DOI: 10.4324/9781003284840-9

and found to be normal. Of course she could have seen through this if she had wanted to.

(p. 375)

Green describes her visit to another ill friend who was recovering from pneumonia. It was election night. Together they heard that Eisenhower won his second term defeating Adlai Stevenson.

> [A]s her friend started to clear the table, Clara, who never liked to be waited on, began to feel very uncomfortable. She said she was feeling too sick to help out and too uncomfortable not to help out, so her friend stopped. They went into the other room to listen to election returns, and Clara said, "if you lie down on that sofa, I'll lie down on this one."
>
> (p. 377)

Soon after she resumed her active schedule, organizing panels, preparing papers, teaching, and attending to her practice. At this stage of life and under these circumstances, Thompson could still give the impression of being impenetrable. In the spring of 1957, she responded to a letter from a friend praising her for her profound clarity:

> I am constantly hearing this and being praised for it. . . . I couldn't become complicated if I tried. Sometimes I wonder if it is really a virtue—it is so easy for me. But that reminds me of something Fromm once said about courage, i.e., we get the ideas that courage is due to a great effort of the will—but most courageous acts are done by people who could not do otherwise—their whole life pattern led them to this point; the next step did not even require conscious decision. I know this has been true of my life. I have lived large areas of it against the culture, but I could not do otherwise, and I cannot put my finger on any one decision. I think there is eternal seeking, and the same is true of my thinking. I just think this way.
>
> (p. 376)

In the summer of 1957, she returned to Provincetown, while many of her students and colleagues attended a symposium on Zen Buddhism and Psychoanalysis sponsored by Erich Fromm's Institute in Mexico City. She too had planned to be present and she missed seeing Fromm's "magnificent estate, high in the hills of Cuernavaca," where peacocks strutted on the lawn (Green, p. 376).

In the winter of 1958, she began to feel weak. Sometime around May, she developed shingles. Green remarks,

> the people who loved her could hardly bear to be close to her at times because they were so touched by the quiet, uncomplaining way in which she suffered the most severe pain.
>
> (p. 376)

By that summer she was back in Provincetown. The shingles persisted. She was unable to take the daily swims that she loved so much. She wrote a dear friend,

> The shingles left me with a neuritis which is dammed uncomfortable, but for the last three days that seems to be greatly improved—so I have high hopes.
>
> (Green, p. 376)

In another letter to her friend she wrote,

> I had three fine days this week and thought it was really over, but yesterday (with the humidity I suppose) it came back again—the itching, I mean. Well, it will surely stop some day, I suppose, and it isn't as bad as it was. I sure am glad it didn't happen during the work year.
>
> (Green, p. 377)

By summer's end, she noticed her liver was enlarged. Some questioned her about why she did not seek medical attention. Her response is sobering: "If it is what I think it is, there's nothing to do" (p. 377). When she did visit her doctor, he told her it was cirrhosis of the liver. Believing him, she began weekly treatments that left her feeling intensely sick. That October, her 65th birthday was not a celebratory event. She seems to have tried to keep up her patient schedule but not her social life. In November of 1958, as Green (1964a) describes it, she wrote to a friend,

> Although I am getting good treatment for it, and they assure me I will get well, I have been forced to greatly reduce my activities, and do you know—I am getting to like being lazy!
>
> (p. 377)

Thompson had hoped she would feel well enough to attend the meetings of the Academy of Psychoanalysis and go on a winter vacation in Antigua. However, soon after one of her treatments, she became ill and bedridden. One rainy Sunday two weeks before her death, her colleague, Nathan Ackerman, visited. "In a hushed voice she told him, I don't suppose there is much hope for this society; we need a change." Clara Thompson "dreamed of a better world and a better way for people to live together" (WAW Newsletter, March 1959, p. 1). In early December, she completed her will, and on December 20, 1958, at the age of 65, she died.

Last Will and Testament

Clara M. Thompson's last will and testament were admitted to probate in New York following her death. It read:

> I Clara Thompson of the county and city of New York, being of sound and disposing mind and memory . . . direct that all my just debts and funeral expenses be paid by my executors. . . . I give and bequeath all my psychoanalytic books pamphlets and reprints which may be in my office, now at 12 east 86th street, New York City . . . to the William Alanson White Institute of Psychiatry, Psychoanalysis and Psychology, chartered under the board of Regents of the State of New York. . . . I give and bequeath all the rest and remainder of my library to my friend, Janet Rioch. . . . I give my jewelry and silverware in equal shares to my nieces Sue Thompson Green and Frances Thompson or the survivors of them. . . . I give to Lillie Fisher who was my maid for thirty years my account in the state mutual building association of Baltimore; and . . . to her my clothing . . . I give to my friend, Miklos Major, of the city of New York, all and any works of art which, at the time of my death, may be in my house situate at 599 Commercial Street Provincetown MA and I give my real property at 599 commercial street to my friends, Philip Malicoat and Barbara Malicoat or to the survivor of them since they love it and helped make it beautiful; and I further give and bequeath to them or to the survivors of them the sum of two thousand dollars. . . . I give to my brother Frank E. Thompson . . . all the rest, residue and remainder.

Sadly, many of the papers she bequeathed to the WAW were lost or damaged in a 2016 flood at the Institute. It is not known what subsequently happened to the library left to her friend Janet Rioch. The silverware and jewelry left to her nieces is untraceable. To Lillie Fisher, she left an unknown sum of money and her clothing. We don't know if that sum was more or less than the $2,000 she left to her friends, the Malicoats.

Our Inheritance—What Clara Thompson Passed on to Us

Leadership

During her tenure as Director of WAWI, Thompson successfully opened training to non-medical clinicians in aligned social science fields. It was a protracted battle that granted access to analytic training at the institute. But there was a limitation. At the conclusion of the same course of study, the non-medical candidates were not granted the same diploma as their medical collogues. Thompson had taken the battle as far as she could.

She had learned many lessons. She cautioned that the nature of psychoanalytic training environments, for better or worse, can resemble families. She warned that within institutes unresolved transferences and countertransference could end in loyalty feuds. Institutes should not become homes from which there is no escape. She argued that graduates should be encouraged to think and act for themselves. Analysts need to see themselves as part of a developing science to which they have a specific contribution to make rather than as members of some isolated group, fanatically loyal. Her words fell mostly on deaf ears.

The Significance of the Analyst

In her pivotal essay, "*Notes on the Psychoanalytic Significance of the Choice of Analyst*" (1938), Thompson affirmed the mutuality of the analytic encounter. She moved the focus of inquiry in psychoanalysis from focusing solely on the patient to the interacting personalities of both patient and analyst. Critical of the analytic theorizing of her time, she wrote:

> If one knew practical psychoanalytic experience only from the papers printed, one might be tempted to assume that the analyst as a personality in reality does not exist and that he never says anything, that he

never leaves the impress of his opinion on the patient in any way that he never makes any mistakes, that, in short, he is not human but a fountain of completely detached wisdom in no way affected personally by anything which goes on.

(p. 205)

She goes on to explain, that

If, on the other hand, one were to believe the anti-psychoanalytic literature, one would see that the patient is completely the victim of the analyst who through suggestion puts ideas into the patient's head which he later analyzes out, the whole process is not necessarily related to the patient's life, but rather to a fantasy in the mind of the analyst.

(p. 206)

She rejects both these views and asserts,

if the analyst does not go so far to completely impose his ideas on the patient, neither is his general attitude towards life in reality of no consequence in the patient's cure or lack of cure.

(p. 206)

In *The Role of the Analyst's Personality in Therapy*,[1] she acknowledges that the analytic situation is more complicated than was initially assumed and gives useful examples of how this is true. She argues that the analyst brings their entire personality to the analytic encounter including their past ways of relating as does the patient. She says:

I believe the patient's interests are best served by analysts who are nonconformists—and certainly not blind conformists—but are always ready to seek new values in the interest of what is good for man. This, of course, puts me in the Sullivanian group. But the Sullivanian orientation did not make me a seeker after truth, no matter where it leads. It only gave me a greater opportunity to develop this aspect of myself. I found the school whose thinking and values approximated what I was seeking for myself.

(Thompson, 1988, p. 130)

Within any discussion of the role of the analysts' personality is the concept of analytic participation and engagement. "This whole effort to understand your own participation and the nature of participation really came from Clara Thompson," says Edgar Levenson in his interview with Hirsch and Iannuzzi (2005, p. 595).

Toxic Identifications

Thompson expanded on Anna Freud's description to further identify the lingering effects of identification with the aggressor on the child's developing personality.[2] As she describes it,

> Since the identification rises primarily out of fear, the child is really joining forces with a hostile power. In doing so he surrenders part of his own interests. He has taken into himself an ideology not because he admires it or believes in it, but chiefly for protective purposes. The enemy he feared from the outside has, so to speak, reappeared inside himself. Toward this incorporated imago the young child has greater difficulty in developing a critical attitude toward the friendly one because any attempt to reject it later tends to rouse the same fear which caused its being accepted in the first place.
>
> (Thompson, 1940, p. 37)

Her clinical concept of identification with the enemy/aggressor and loss of the sense of self and the lingering effects have been seamlessly woven into psychoanalytic work without so much as a nod to Thompson's stellar 1940 essay. So too is the concept in her essay "Dutiful Child' Resistance" (1931) that paved the way for this understanding of how toxic parents are internalized and inhibit emotional and social development. She explains,

> The child unable to cope with hostility directed toward them by their parents may renounce his own interests for the sake of peace and take over his parent's attitudes.
>
> (Thompson, 1940, p. 38)

Thompson's ideas appear in the work of later interpersonal/relational analysts. For example, when Levenson (1990) says,

> I think there is a reality of experience which is obscured—not because that is the nature of experience—but because the patient's version of his

or her life has been distorted, literally twisted out of shape, by the vicissi-
tudes of interpersonal anxiety. The patient's vision of life is full of inatten-
tions, repressions, distortions because that constricted vision is necessary
to survival, by not mobilizing the anxiety of the person's caretakers.

(p. 299)

Providing a New Experience

Thompson taught the importance of providing the patient with a new experience and offered detailed clinical examples of the creation of that experience as result of the openness and directness of the analyst. She pointed to
ways of interacting that do not depend on words,

> We must relate to the patient with more than our intellects. We feel
> things that sometimes do not reach the level of verbal awareness. For
> example, why do I frequently yawn with a certain patient, why do I feel
> restless with another, and vaguely annoyed at times with a third? Is it
> simply the time of day or my state of weariness, or is there some more
> serious failure of communication? In the case of the yawning, I discov-
> ered in one case that it was especially frequent when a strong parasitic
> (dependent) clinging tendency was predominant during the hour. We
> both found that this was useful clue that the hour seemed to be getting
> nowhere, and that it actually was more effective in altering her attitude
> than direct statement would have been. Undoubtedly yawning can mean
> different things in different situations. (Thompson, (1988c) p. 120-130).

Wolstein (1982) built on Thompson's position arguing that unconscious
experience,

> Includes both the processes of unique individuality and the patterns of
> shareable identity of the particular psychoanalyst and patient, as either
> or both transform and translate unconscious into conscious psychic
> experience during their coparticipant therapeutic inquiry.

(Wolstein, p. 416)

In Benjamin Wolstein's interview with Irwin Hirsch (2000), he confirms
how influenced he was by his analysis with Thompson. He says,

> My major influence, obviously, was Clara Thompson. I'll always have
> deep affection and regard for her. She took me on a trip and I took her

on a trip. It was a quest for psychic freedom, you know. In that context, anything went. Of course, we had differences of opinion; I mean, about the question of countertransference and how to work with it. This made our differences real. She used to take the established position of the early 1950s— "that belongs in my analysis, not in yours." Of course, I was a bit of a wiseacre. I used to ask her, "if it belongs in your analysis, what is it doing in mine?" She didn't get defensive about it. She laughed. And eventually, something I'll always respect her for, we began to do a certain amount of open analysis. I began to realize how her psychology actually affected some of the work that went on between us. And I thought that was extraordinary for the time . . .

(pp. 187–188)

Thompson possessed "therapeutic courage." It is an underutilized term in psychoanalytic work but one that is immensely important. It takes courage to be with someone—to expose your feelings, thoughts, and actions, and to witness the same in a reciprocal process. That is at the core of Thompson's psychotherapeutic process.

Poignantly, at the conclusion of Wolstein's analysis, he gave Thompson a string of pearls. He lovingly referred to that fact and added that she requested to be buried wearing those pearls (D'Ercole, 2017), perhaps it was a symbol of their enduring connection.

Women's Psychology: A Cultural View

Drawing from sociology, anthropology, psychoanalysis, and other social sciences Thompson formulated a culture-based understanding of the psychology of women. Her clinical views of women were developed through and limited by the lens of the culture at the time. She was a part of a critical period when liberal scientists in America were challenging racial and sexual boundaries. As Wake (2011) suggests, her cohort of social science colleagues began to question universal notions of "normal" and "abnormal." For these cross-disciplinary professionals, "modernity was about the recognition that ambiguity, rather than clear-cut categories, was where all understanding begins" (p. 4). Wake finds that as Thompson and others in her cohort wrestled with these boundaries, a contradiction between public and private liberalism widened.

Thompson was not unaware of her theoretical limitations. She recognized that what she offered was, as she put it, a "limited but very significant view of the situation" (Thompson, 1941, p. 1). She was right on both counts. It was significant because it was a departure from an understanding of personality development that was biologically driven yet limited by a reliance on binary categories of gender and sexuality. She embraced the concept of culture to correct distorted views about the nature of women in her time. She never makes grand or sweeping pronouncements but rather focuses on what she knows through her own experience and that of her patients.

Agreements and Divergence

Thompson was in a dialogue with her colleagues, beginning with Ferenczi and later Horney, Sullivan, and Fromm. While they worked together, they each made substantive modifications to each other's ideas. To borrow from Stern (2010), they were partners in thought.

Thompson was a non-conformist even in ideas. She disagreed with Ferenczi, who believed the analyst needed to activate the reliving of traumatic childhood experiences. She felt strongly that the psychoanalytic situation itself would bring about regressive behavior, and therefore the analyst should not intensify that experience but meet it when it occurs. She also disagreed with Ferenczi's position on the need for and use of love in the analytic relationship. She believed his definition of love was shortsighted. Instead of offering as Ferenczi did, a non-sexual passion (love), she felt what patients needed more of was respect. It's possible that advocating for respect over love was more aligned with her personality—influenced by her reserved New England roots. However, she did believe that patients who were not loved as children could not metabolize or take in love when it was offered; instead, she warned, they might use it to manipulate the analyst. Her ideas were more consistent with budding theories on the use of an object and early patterns of character development.

With respect to interpersonal theory, Thompson gave more weight to the influence of her psychoanalytic ancestors than did Sullivan, who insisted that his theory was unique and not heavily reliant on past theorists. She was less committed to his sharp division between psychoanalysis and interpersonal theory (Sullivan, 1953). She believed Sullivan left no room for change in his model of self. She agreed with Erich Fromm that Sullivan's concept of the self was an expression of the dominant alienated social character (Thompson, 1956). Thompson thought Sullivan had limited his field of observation to man's attempt to fit into our specific society and that he did not concern himself with unrealized potential, with what one might become in different circumstances. Because of this limitation, she stated, Sullivan "has only vague things to say about maturity. . . . He has practically nothing to say about mature love. He does define what passes for love at the juvenile and preadolescent levels."

In contrast, Fromm, she notes, is more concerned with the "problem of maturity" and how the individual may succeed in transcending their culture (Thompson, 1964b, p. 99).

Thompson disagreed with Horney and Fromm on their essentialist notions of female psychology, arguing instead that biological functions do not surpass the demands placed on the individual by society. While she leaned more in the direction of Fromm's thinking, her feminism took issue with certain of his ideas—women's sexual needs and the notion that if women adopted more masculine characteristics, men would become angrier because they need women to take care of them.

Among her other analytic legacies, Thompson clarified the significance of the analyst, the role of their personality, and how toxic identifications can shape personality. She underscored the importance of providing a new experience in the analytic encounter, one that was more empathic and genuine. She left us a culturalist view of the psychology of women that pointed to the connection of individual psychology with the injustices in society.

Thompson's Psychoanalytic Family Tree

Ernst Falzeder (2015) hypothesizes the notion of the enduring aspects of the psychoanalytic family tree. He maintains,

> Through the training analysis, each psychoanalyst becomes part of a genealogy that ultimately goes back to Sigmund Freud and a handful of early pioneers. Evidently, each training and supervising analyst has her or his own theoretical and practical preferences, with which the analysands are confronted and by which they are deeply influenced.
>
> (p. 77)

Falzeder accounts for the influence of a "sibling" peer group of fellow candidates, as he traces the genealogy of the psychoanalytic family, thus outlining a psychoanalytic lineage that extends over decades with intersecting branches.

In this psychoanalytic family tree, Clara Thompson is linked by one degree of separation to Freud through his direct descendant, Sándor Ferenczi.

Thompson trained and mentored the preeminent analysts of the first two generations of Interpersonal Psychoanalysts,[3] including Edgar Levenson, Ruth Moulton, Ruth Lesser, Ralph Crowley, Lewis Hill, Erwin Singer, Edward Tauber, Benjamin Wolstein, and others. Among her analysands were Steven Adrian, Kate Frankenthal, Emmanuel Ghent, Maurice R. Green, Lewis Hill, Bernie Kalinkowitz, Ruth Lesser, Ruth Moulton, Rose Spiegel, Bertram Schaffner, Harry Stack Sullivan, and Benjamin Wolstein.

As Wolstein noted,

> I had to consider the possibility of some sort of generational transmission from Ferenczi's "dialogue of unconscious" to Thompson's "direct psychoanalytic experience" to my "experiential field of therapy."
>
> (p. 189)

Another analysand, Ruth Lesser had "enormous respect, gratitude and affection" for Clara Thompson, her daughter, Dr. Judy Lesser recalled.[4] It is worth noting that Ruth Lesser was doubly influenced by Thompson's rethinking of the fundamental tenets of psychoanalysis and Fromm's sociopolitical conceptualizations. Lesser (1992) explains how she appreciated the richness of her time in supervision with Fromm. He taught her that no two people were alike and that the analyst achieves an understanding of the patient by allowing herself/himself to be "soaked with the individual patient's feelings" while "being aware of his/her own capacity for similar experiences" (p. 483).

This interactiveness of experience is underscored time and again by Thompson's heirs. For example, Levenson (2005) clarified a component of experience:

> There's something all therapists do and essentially I think it is to get involved in a deconstruction of the patient's narrative. Whenever the patient tells you the story of his or her life, you either expand it by free association or by a detailed inquiry. In the process of working through,

I think the patient is getting better, not because your metapsychology works, but because somewhere in that process you're doing a real deconstructive inquiry. The detailed inquiry isn't intended to make it all clearer, but to open things up: to unpack the story in such a way that it gets more complicated and more enriched and more interesting, clinically. Now it seems to me that what happens at that point makes a significant difference because patients are then more open to reorganizing their experience.

(p. 598)

Levenson (2003) concludes, "It seems likely that the inquiry *is* the therapeutic act; that as Marshall Mcluhan put it, the medium *is* indeed the message (p. 233).

WAWI and the NYU Postdoctoral Program (NYU Postdoc)

There is a close connection between WAWI and NYU Postdoc because of Clara Thompson. The history between WAWI and NYU Postdoc began in 1952 when a group of "matriculants" from WAWI were feeling unsure about the Institute's commitment to training psychologists as Aron (1996) explains. They submitted a proposal to establish a postdoctoral program in psychoanalysis at New York University. The psychologists in this group included Bernie Kalinkowitz, Erwin Singer, and Avrum Ben-Avi (p. 4).

Upon approval of the proposal, it was Clara Thompson's analysands who assumed administrative leadership; Bernie Kalinkowitz became the first Director, and Ruth Lesser, the Clinic Director. They each left an indelible mark on what would come to be called, the New York University, Postdoctoral Program in Psychotherapy and Psychoanalysis.

NYU Postdoc remains the only psychoanalytic training program located within a university. Esther Menaker, who was in a study group with Thompson, taught the first course in the program (personal communication, 1992). NYU Postdoc was dedicated to welcoming psychologists and other PhD-level mental health professionals for analytic training and provided an environment of academic freedom, encouraging diverse points of view. Courses with Freudian, Sullivanian, Interpersonal-Humanistic and Frommian perspectives were offered. A course on Clara Thompson's contributions was absent. Within a decade, theoretical divisions became apparent, leading to the formation of a two-track system: Freudian and

Interpersonal-Humanistic. Aron (1996) explains that the "I-H" hyphenation represented "Sullivan's theoretical legacy," combined with the term Fromm had applied to his own outlook, "Humanistic," thus the I-H track (p. 6). While there are many versions of the story of the evolution of the track system at NYU Postdoc, the one with which I am most familiar involves a series of disputes over the place of object relations theory within the program. It amounted to a showdown between Ruth Lesser and Bernard Friedland over a course in object relations. Emmanuel Ghent, another of Thompson's analysands, spearheaded the move to establish a Relational track. Some of the first and second-generation Interpersonal psychoanalysts who trained at WAWI (e.g., Philip Bromberg, Darlene Ehrenberg, Stephen Mitchell, and Donnel Stern (to name only a few)) affiliated with the relational track while others remained with the I-H track (e.g., Wolstein, Levenson, and others).

From Interpersonal to Relational

While Thompson, Sullivan, Fromm, and Fromm-Reichmann revised classical psychoanalytic theory. Together and separately, the shaped their visions of psychoanalysis. They each ascribed to the continuous and inevitable mutual unconscious influence between analyst and patient. Subsequent generations of interpersonal theorists continued this thesis as they elaborated a diverse set of concepts, including empathy, spontaneity, mutuality, a feminist gender analysis, a culturalist and field theory view of the psychoanalytic encounter and reappraisals of sexual and gender identities. Sometimes known as the American school, interpersonal psychoanalysis's early pioneers played a critical role in incorporating a gender analysis, attributing the difficulties in women's lives to social conditions and made fledgling attempts to consider the effects of systemic racism on human experience.[5]

Interpersonal psychoanalysis is part of the foundation of relational psychoanalysis. While both Thompson and Sullivan used the term "interpersonal," the early use of the term "relational" can be traced to a series of papers from 1969 through 1988 by Thompson's analysand, Gerald Chrzanowski. In "Implications of Interpersonal Theory" (1973), later published as "Sullivan's Concept of Malevolent Transformation (A Symposium)—Malevolent transformation and the Negative Therapeutic Reaction" (1978), Chrzanowski notes the "relational field" of development and "relational patterns" of experience and layers of anxiety (Chrzanowski, 1978, p. 406).

Unraveling what is interpersonal from what is relational is a complicated undertaking that may not yield much in the way of results argues Stern (2006). He explains there is an unresolvable problem attached to untangling the relationship between each school of thought.

> Interpersonal and Relational psychoanalysis are large theories, umbrella theories, so that there is often as much disagreement within them as there is between them. The only answers to the question of how to untangle the relationship of the two theories with one another are the answers of individuals, and even then, the answers depend on context. Sometimes the context is primarily theoretical or scholarly, sometimes a matter of personal commitment, and sometimes a political or even moral issue.
>
> (p. 565)

He identifies

> A number of the "most prominent Relational writers (Philip Bromberg, Darlene Ehrenberg, Emmanuel Ghent, Jay Greenberg, Stephen Mitchell), three of whom were also among the original five members of the faculty of the Relational Track (Bromberg, Bernard Friedland, Ghent, Jim Fosshage, Mitchell) at the New York University Postdoctoral Program in Psychotherapy and Psychoanalysis (NYU Postdoc), did their psychoanalytic training at the White Institute, a psychoanalytic training program with a comparative bent, but very much the home of Interpersonal psychoanalysis.
>
> (p. 565)

Stern and Hirsch (2017a; Stern, 2017) identify relatively unknown second- and third-generation interpersonal analysts who nonetheless made significant contributions to the analytic literature from the 1930s to the 1970s as well as recent analysts who have contributed to the interpersonal tradition (pp. 1–3).

In the late 1960s, the psychoanalyst Ruth Moulton began to write articles on women informed by a modified "Thompsonian perspective" (see

"A Survey and Reevaluation of the Concept of Penis Envy," (Moulton, 1970). Later, she wrote:

> Thinking about women, one must go back briefly to the accepted theories that existed when Horney started to write. Freud had written very little directly about female sexual development. His "Three Essays on Sexuality" (1905) were primarily based on observations about men; women were seen as secondary with no unique identity of their own. This can be explained by the fact that his early female patients were mostly hysterics full of sexual inhibitions and tied up in Oedipal struggles and strong transferences to him as "the father"; they were therefore not very good subjects for the study of normal sexual development.
>
> (Moulton, 1975, p. 207)

Since the publication of the Ferenczi diary in 1988, speculation swirled around the subject of whether Thompson was sexually abused by her father. No precise data can be provided to support the initial statement contained in Ferenczi's diary. The conclusion based on those lines is at best speculative and most likely as Dupont (D'Ercole, 2022) suggests a mixing of patients to maintain anonymity.

Thompson did not adopt all of Ferenczi's ideas into her work. As she made clear, she "discarded" some of them. She was cautious about the use of regression to facilitate recall and she did not focus specifically on childhood sexual trauma and its effects in adults. However, she was not afraid to know herself. In a footnote (Thompson, 1988c) she advocates for continuing analysis in supervision:

> I have participated in a small seminar of graduates in which the emphasis is entirely on countertransference problems. It is a kind of miracle club, in which the participants swear the patient must have been listening in, because he reacts so often as predicted to the insight gained by the analyst. Should we not all subject this delicate, sensitive instrument—our own personality—to frequent overhauling! I do not mean necessarily extensive analysis but checking on the spots where things are not going smoothly, especially with our patients. We do this as a matter of course with our cars, radios, microscopes—why not with the most delicate instrument of all—ourselves!
>
> (p. 130)

A Perfect Leader for Her Time

Fromm's (1964) *Foreword* to Thompson's collected papers pays tribute to her importance to so many people and to her extensive impact on the field. He claimed, "[S]he was a leader for the time."

> A rare person who could take a leading role in the formation of an independent psychoanalytic group and continue to guide it . . . she was a thoroughly independent person, averse to rules and principles with which she did not agree; at the same time she did not endow her own theoretical principles with a halo that would make her fight all others.
>
> (p. vi)

Thompson encouraged her students to find their own analytic voice rather than copying hers—an admirable approach, although not one that would create a brand.

This biography, follows work of Clara Thompson, drawing on the oral history tradition. Toward that end, I have included several moving eulogies. This one was delivered on December 24, 1958; in it Meyer Maskin spoke of her essence and of his love for her.

> Grief is a lonely marauder, like a stabbing, unsharable pain. What can be done with words to lament an absence, an anguish in one's body, dusty memories.
>
> What can one do but drone repetitively . . . endlessly . . . incredulously: Clara is dead . . . dead . . . Clara is dead . . .
>
> In the ebb of grief we mourn for ourselves, for the massive fragments of ourselves that disappear with our interred friends.
>
> If anyone still clings to the illusion of himself as some self-contained domain, let him discover in mourning how uncontained he really is, as his grieving self is inexorably drained like sand running out of an hour-glass chamber.
>
> I detest eulogies . . . contrived sequences of selected and wistful adjectives which describe what human beings can never be. I want only to talk about Clara as I knew her and experienced her . . . so that what I am . . . here and now . . . is partly Clara, for she was my teacher and therapist and friend.
>
> How else, indeed, shall we estimate a person, save for what his existence has yielded to another? What is more terrifying than that our living shall have made no difference to anyone?

That Clara lived has meant to me that dignity and courage are living actions and not words selected for an obituary.

She endured profound personal tragedy and tormenting pain in such good grace and with such undemonstrative forbearance that—unless one knew the bitter facts themselves, one would have presumed that her life had been simple, careless and carefree.

And yet it was Clara's agony to lose her beloved prematurely and to endure a protracted physical dying in a state of utter mental lucidity.

Clara made living appear so damnably simple. As if it were perfectly routine for a young lady of 19th century upbringing and of New England biblical rearing to become a physician . . . and a psychiatrist of all things . . . to go off on jaunts alone to unlikely Budapest without a word of Hungarian . . . and to metamorphose as a psychoanalyst in an era when most people had hardly heard of the word . . . or if they had, reacted to it with derision. Or to live in open and unabashed affection and love with a man, legally unable to marry her . . . and to do this without self-consciousness, self-commiseration . . . or, for that matter without the belligerence and defiance and the exhibitionistic self-adulation of the professional feminists and bohemians.

Years before the pretentious and self-conscious avant-gardists flocked to Provincetown, Clara summered there in a modified fishhouse, immersed in the simplicity of wind, sun and sea . . . and cooked goulash. For the amazing quality which characterized Clara is that she lived a fantastically non-conformist life . . . that is to say, she lived her own personal life without using it to diminish others. She made no raucous cult of individuality and creativity; she did not stridently shout "Down with the bourgeoisie" or underscore comparisons between her own rebelliousness and the conventional submissiveness of others. She quietly set her own course, sought he own destiny as a woman and lacked the need to indoctrinate or impress others. Here, surely was Clara's divine touch: her awareness of the incredible diversity among people . . . of their authentic need for different ways of living. . . . And hence Clara could, without sacrificing her own style of life, respond appreciatively to such different, heterogenous types and do it with such unassuming simplicity and directness, that each person was likely to feel, in his own egotism, that surely she preferred his unique brand to all others. Here was the secret of Clara's powers of reassurance . . . of her talent to function like a gyroscope in human groups, maintaining a steady center of gravity in the tower of Babel. Her strength and authority issued not from any need for power or possession or from some need to convert others into her own image . . . but from an authentic belief in the genuine differences among people and he need to foster and preserve this diversity.

No one that I have known had a more varied group of acquaintances and friends. Some of whom heartily disliked each other, but each of whom could converse with Clara. For the charm of an encounter with Clara was that one could disagree with her, dispute, criticize . . . without evoking resentment or rancor. With Clara, one could live in comfortable disagreement . . . and even like oneself for disagreeing.

I could tease her, joke with her, satirize her . . . and, as is true only of the genuinely strong, never need to worry about hurting her.

As I perceived her, her primary weakness was a too ready giving to and forgiving of the weak, the lost, the excommunicated. In her need to protect and to provide for the weak . . . leaving the strong to shift for themselves . . . Clara overlooked the substantial contribution she could have made to the strong, as well. Too often, she was a living Miss Lonely Hearts whose compassion gained her contempt.

Clara had a sharp, sure grasp of the spurious masquerading as the real . . . of the empty verbalism posing for the deed. With devastating accuracy, she could summarize a personality in three terse sentences . . . and the same, unpretentious clarity is evident in her luminous writing which avoids the dialogue of ambiguity and fatuity that characterize so much of psychoanalytic writings.

There are few people, I'm sure, who, knowing Clara as long as I have, will not remain grateful for her plain down-right goodness, administered with principle and tact. Twenty odd years ago, in the midst of the Depression, when all the training analysts to whom I was referred responded with some enthusiasm to me until they discovered that I happened to be broke . . . and then each thought it would be a fine thing for some other colleague to grant me a partial scholarship, Clara alone was so bountiful in her financial arrangements, and withal so casual and disarming about it all . . . that I found myself an analytic student almost before I realized what was happening. As a matter of fact, she once loaned me some money to take a course I could ill afford, and salved my pride by suggesting that I could repay her by letting her read my notes. For her pains, she was later accused by a not so generous colleague of running an espionage service. When I was on leave during the war . . . restless, angry, disconsolate, Clara decided it would be good for me to have a vacation in Provincetown . . . and God alone knows how . . . arranged for a car and gasoline to cart an ungrateful soldier there.

And when my wife died, it was Clara who repeatedly . . . completely ignoring my irritability and my rebuffs . . . kept inviting me for dinner and letting me talk out all the sad talk that was choking me. And, when I felt better, she deftly withdrew her aids and props . . . as if they had never been there.

This fantastic tact she had of somehow appearing when needed and disappearing when not needed . . . this was her glory but bereft of power . . . for she never made one feel indebted. I don't know how she did it. . . . I wish only I could say that I had always been as generous to her as she had been to me. Mostly I learned from Clara to develop courage out of conviction. And, when years ago, as a young analytic student, I was drowning in a fountain of psychoanalytic verbiage, it was from Clara I learned that the continental accents who quoted Freud so loquaciously were not necessarily making sense . . . that psychoanalysis was only beginning and that an ultimate truth was yet to be spoken.

In the clear autonomy of her ways, Clara had no trouble departing form the advantages and honorariums that were readily available to her within the established church of orthodox psychoanalysis, to pursue a psychiatry of good sense and good will.

In a time of tawdry angry men, self-proclaimed howlers, outsiders, prophets and rebels, heaping fad upon cult and sect upon egotism, I find Clara to be the most genteel, civilized rebel I have ever known, who sought the cool freedom of undefiant, uncompetitive, authentic disagreement as the sole realistic basis for people living with people . . .

Hence no dogma will ever perpetuate Clara's memory as no words will contain her. Loneliness and tears will bear evidence that Clara is dead. As best I could, I loved Clara. That she lived augmented me. . . . Her death diminishes me.

(Maskin, 1958, Eulogy)

Has Clara M. Thompson Really Disappeared?

For years I have felt compelled to tell the story of the life of Clara M. Thompson. It is now clear to me that this story of Thompson's life is also about my journey in psychoanalysis. By working closely with the analysands and students of Clara Thompson, I experienced a part of her that has persisted.

Thompson's legacy is most palpably felt in her encounters with others. Beyond her written word, which is significant in a truly interpersonal tradition, she left an imprint that is carried from one person to the next, through generations.

This story of her life relies heavily on her voice—through her letters, interviews, her writing, and the words of those of her analysand, colleagues, students, and friends. They say how powerfully they felt her connection to them and how she shaped their clinical work. They each attest to her positive human qualities as well as her defensive diffidence. She was generous, she recognized the constraints imposed by society. She was the quintessential interpersonalist, always attuned to the mutuality of the encounter.

Thompson entered the field of psychoanalysis on the ground floor. Her treatment and collaboration with Ferenczi broadened her views to include his notion of the continuous and mutually interacting nature of the practice of psychoanalysis. While she did not endorse Ferenczi's use of regression as a trauma-informed approach to treatment, she did concur with many of his other ideas, specifically the central importance of empathy, authenticity, spontaneity, respect, and tenderness—essentially human ingredients in an effective therapeutic process. Those ideas were further refined and expanded upon under the influence of Harry Stack Sullivan and Erich Fromm—and to some degree Karen Horney—who added a new perspective to the concept of anxiety in personality formation and the social context of development. The early influence of the Women's Missionary Society and the Women's Suffragist Movement (see *Clara M. Thompson's Early Years and Professional Awakening: An American Psychoanalyst (1893–1933)*) was woven into her ideas about the psychology of women. By drawing from her own experiences as a woman, she refined and developed a cultural analysis of the problems women faced in society. Her role as leader of the William Alanson White Institute consumed the last decade of her life.

What we come to really know about Thompson on these pages is only a segment of a robust and complex life. My hope was that this biographical narrative would draw a detailed and fuller picture of this courageous psychoanalytic pioneer. Thompson's life and work were uncannily prescient. She pioneered a life as a woman largely unfettered by conventional norms. As a psychiatrist and psychoanalyst, she broke boundaries, reevaluated orthodox psychoanalysis integrated it with discoveries from the budding social sciences, and wove it together with her distinctly American pragmatism.

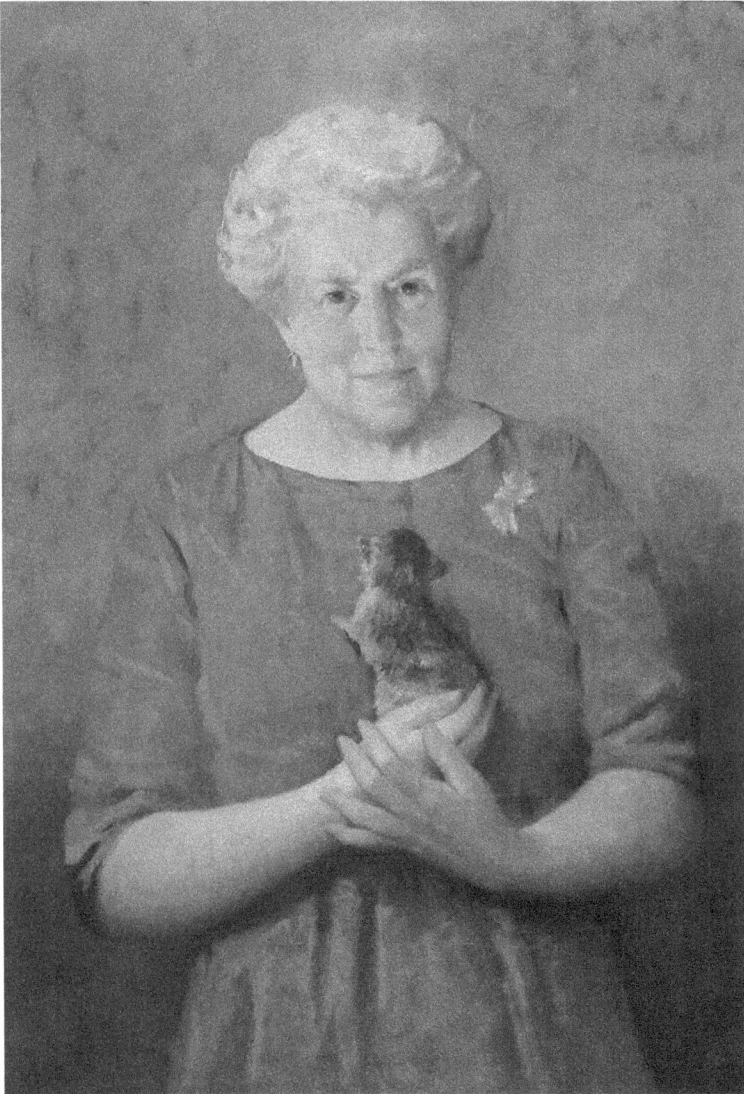

Figure 8.1 Clara Thompson with her cat. Original artist unknown. Reprinted with permission, © William Alanson White Institute.

She transformed her early proclaimed religious mission to save souls, to the relief of human suffering, and to improving the quality of lives. Her new form of psychoanalysis was foundational, first to the interpersonal and then relational psychoanalytic schools. It is time now to not only resurrect the

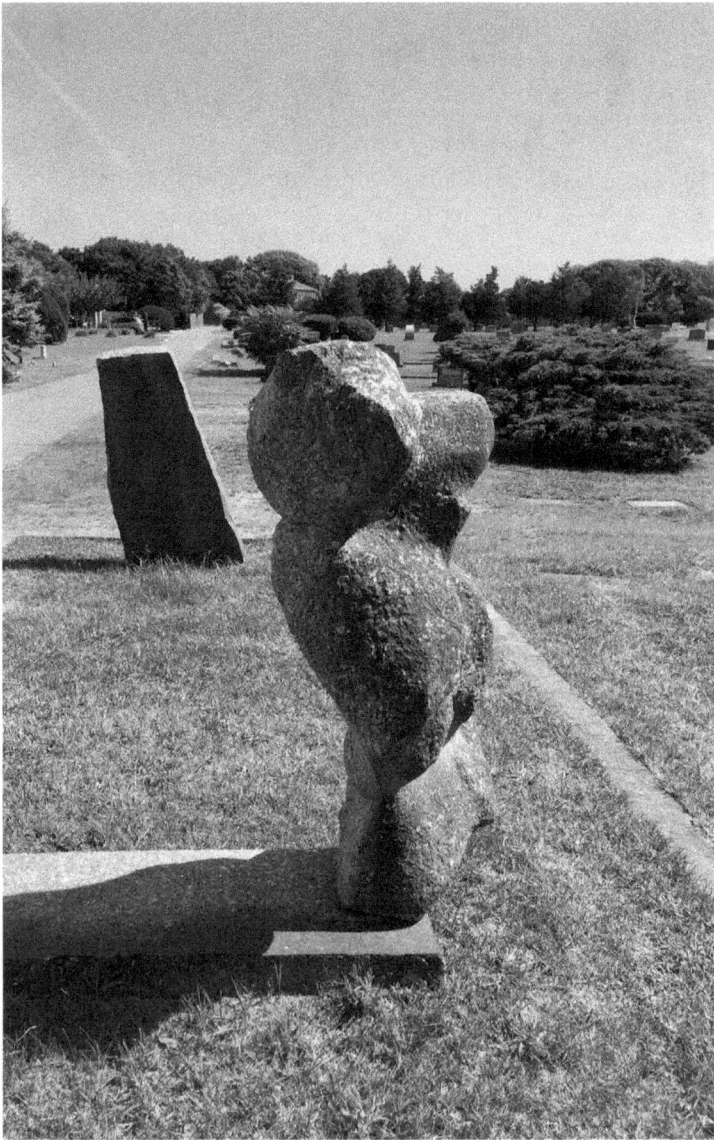

Figure 8.2 Clara Thompson and Henry Major's graves, Provincetown; photo by David Mamo.

oral history of Thompson but also reexamine and preserve her written word as we move ahead with contemporary psychoanalytic thought.

As the political poet Adrienne Rich (1986) might argue, remembering Thompson's accomplishments as a woman of the 20th century is an act of "resisting amnesia." As one of the many hidden, accomplished women of the 20th century, it behooves us to look and see what she achieved, where and why she fell short, and how close she came to touching the future. Her life is a model for taking personal and professional risks.

It is time to recognize Thompson's scholarly contributions, to acknowledge the force of her passion for goodwill and kindness, to appreciate how she accomplished establishing a place for herself despite social prejudices, and to acknowledge the many lives she touched and those she made better along the way.

Notes

1 This paper was originally published in 1956 in the *American Journal of Psychotherapy*, *10*(2), 347–359.
2 The concept of identification with the aggressor was originally described by Anna Freud in *The Ego and Mechanisms of Defence* by Anna Freud (A. Freud, 1937).
3 While many people are referenced in these letters, I've made only a modest attempt to discover what role they may have played at the William Alanson White Institute. The early interpersonal literature is vast, stellar, and exceedingly influential as, Stern et al. (1995) have demonstrated in their edited collection, *Pioneers of Interpersonal Psychoanalysis*. For additional essays, see the edited volume by Lionells et al., *Handbook of interpersonal psychoanalysis* (1995). Also, E. Witenberg, *Psychoanalysis today* (1973). E. Witenberg (Ed.), *Interpersonal explorations in psychoanalysis: New Directions in theory and practice*. New York: Basic Books.
4 Lesser's daughter recalls the story of her mother even brought her young daughter to sessions with Thompson. The child would sit in the waiting area. (Personal communication, Judy Lesser, 11/21/2021).
5 I refer the reader to the work of both early pioneers and subsequent second- and third-generation interpersonalists, in Stern et al. (1995); Lionells et al. (1995); and Stern and Hirsch (2017).
   Letter from Clara Thompson to Ralph Crawley. The Oskar Diethelm library, DeWitt Wallace institute for the history of psychiatry. The Weill Cornell Medical College, The Ralph Crowley Papers, Box 5, Fol. 7., New York, NY.

References

Aron, L. (1996) *A meeting of minds: Mutuality in psychoanalysis*. Routledge Press, New York.

Chrzanowski, G. (1973). Implications of interpersonal theory. In E. G. Witenberg (Ed.), *Interpersonal explorations in psychoanalysis: New directions in theory and practice* (pp. 132–146). New York: Basic Books.

Chrzanowski, G. (1978). Malevolent transformation and the negative therapeutic reaction. *Contemporary Psychoanalysis*, *14*(3), 405–414.

D'Ercole, A. (2017). On finding Clara Thompson. *Contemporary Psychoanalysis*, *53*(1), 63–68.

D'Ercole, A. (2022). *Clara M. Thompson's early years and professional awakening: An American psychoanalyst (1893–1933)*. New York: Routledge Press.

Falzeder, E. (2015). *Psychoanalytic filiations: Mapping the psychoanalytic movement*. London: Karnac Books.

Freud, Anna: *The Ego and the Mechanisms of Defence*. London: Hogarth Press, 1937.

Fromm, E. (1964). Foreword. (p. v, vi.) In M. R. Green (Ed.), *Interpersonal psychoanalysis: The selected papers of Clara M. Thompson* (pp. v–vi). New York: Basic Books.

Freud, S. (1905) Three essays on sexuality. The Standard Edition of the Complete Psychological Works of Sigmund Freud,7(1901–1905). A case of Hysteria, Three essays on sexuality and other works, 123–246.

Green, M. R. (1964a). Her life. (p. 347–377). In M. R. Green (Ed.), *Interpersonal psychoanalysis: The selected papers of Clara M. Thompson*. New York: Basic Books.

Green, M. R. (1964b). *Interpersonal psychoanalysis: The selected papers of Clara M. Thompson*. New York: Basic Books.

Hirsch, I. (2000). Interview with Benjamin Wolstein. *Contemporary Psychoanalysis, 36*(2), 187–232.

Lesser, R. (1992). Frommian therapeutic practice: "A few rich hours." *Contemporary Psychoanalysis*, *28*, 483–494.

Levenson, E. A. (1990). Reply to Hoffman. *Contemporary Psychoanalysis*, *26*, 299–304.

Levenson, E. A. (2003). On seeing what is said: Visual aids in the psychoanalytic process. *Contemporary Psychoanalysis*, *39*, 233–249.

Levenson, E. A. (2005). Response to commentaries. *Contemporary Psychoanalysis*, *41*(4), 749–750.

Levenson, E. A., Hirsch, I., & Iannuzzi, V. (2005). Interview with Edgar A. Levenson January 24, 2004. *Contemporary Psychoanalysis*, *41*(4), 593–644.

Lionells, M., Fiscalini, J., Mann, C. M., & Stern, D. B. (1995). *The handbook of interpersonal psychoanalysis*. Hillsdale, NJ: Analytic Press.

Maskin, M. (1958). In memoriam: Clara Thompson, 1893–1958, unpublished eulogy.

Moulton, R. (1970). A survey and reevaluation of the concept of penis envy. *Contemporary Psychoanalysis, 7*(1), 84–104.

Moulton, R. (1975). Early papers on women: Horney to Thompson. *American Journal of Psychoanalysis, 35*(3), 207–223.

Rich, A. (1986). *Blook, bread, and poetry, selected prose: Resisting amnesia: History and personal life.* New York: Norton & Company.

Stern, D. (2006) States of relatedness. Are ideas part of the family? *Contemporary Psychoanalysis, 42*(4), 565–576

Stern, D. (2010) *Partners in thought: Working with unformulated experience, dissociation and enactment.* Routledge Press, New York. https://doi.org/10.4324/9780203880388

Stern, D. B. (2017). Introduction: "The history of the William Alanson White Institute" by Clara Thompson. *Contemporary Psychoanalysis, 53*(1), 1–6.

Stern, D. B., & Hirsch, I. (2017). *The interpersonal perspective in psychoanalysis, 1960s–1990s: Rethinking transference and countertransference.* Oxon, Ox and New York: Routledge Press.

Sullivan, H. S. (1953). *The interpersonal theory of psychiatry.* New York: W. W. Norton & Company.

Thompson, C. (1931). "Dutiful child" resistance. *Psychoanalytic Review, 18*(4), 426–433.

Thompson, C. (1938). Notes on the psychoanalytic significance of the choice of analyst. *Psychiatry, I*, 205–216.

Thompson, C. (1940). Identification with the enemy and loss of the sense of self. *Psychoanalytic Quarterly, 9*(1), 37–50.

Thompson, C. (1941). The role of women in this culture. *Psychiatry, 4*(1), 1–8.

Thompson, C. M. (1988a). The role of the analyst's personality in therapy. *Essential Papers On Countertransference, ed. by B. Wolstein, New York (New York University Press) 1988, pp. 120–130.*

Thompson, C. (1988b). Sullivan and Fromm. In M. R. Green (Ed.), *Interpersonal psychoanalysis: The selected papers of Clara M. Thompson* (pp. 95–100). New York: Basic Books.

Thompson, C. (1988c). Sándor Ferenczi, 1873–1933. *Contemporary Psychoanalysis, 24*, 182–195.

Wake, N. (2011). *Private practices: Harry Stack Sullivan, the science of homosexuality, and American liberalism.* New Brunswick, NJ: Rutgers University Press.

Wolstein, B. (1982). The psychoanalytic theory of unconscious psychic experience. *Contemporary Psychoanalysis, 18*, 412–437.

Index

Note: Page numbers in *italics* indicate a figure on the corresponding page.

For Product Safety Concerns and Information please contact our EU
representative GPSR@taylorandfrancis.com
Taylor & Francis Verlag GmbH, Kaufingerstraße 24, 80331 München, Germany

9 781032 257532